Clinical Sports Medicine

Clinical Sports Medicine

Edited by

Robert C. Cantu, M.D.
Chief, Neurosurgery Service
Director, Service of Sports Medicine
Emerson Hospital
Concord, Massachusetts

THE COLLAMORE PRESS
D.C. Heath and Company
Lexington, Massachusetts
Toronto

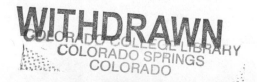

Copyright © 1984 by D.C. Heath and Company

All rights reserved. No part of this publication may be reproduced or transmitted in any form or by any means, electronic or mechanical, including photocopy, recording, or any information storage or retrieval system, without permission in writing from the publisher.

Published simultaneously in Canada

Printed in the United States of America

International Standard Book Number: 0-669-06842-X

Library of Congress Catalog Card Number: 83-71035

Library of Congress Cataloging in Publication Data

Clinical sports medicine.

   Papers presented at the Annual Meeting of the New England Chapter of the American College of Sports Medicine, Nov. 19–20, 1982.
   Includes bibliographical references and index.
   1. Sports medicine—Congresses. I. Cantu, Robert C. II. American College of Sports Medicine. New England Chapter. Meeting (1982: Emerson Hospital) [DNLM: 1. Sports medicine—Congresses. QT 260 C641 1982]
RC1201.C57   1984   617'.1027   83–71035
ISBN 0–669–06842–X

Contents

	Acknowledgments	vii
	Contributing Authors	ix
Part I.	*Predicting Sports Performance*	1
Chapter 1.	**Check Your Talent, Choose Your Sport** *David G. Watson, M.B.B.S.*	3
Chapter 2.	**Anthropometric, Physiologic, and Psychological Measures to Predict Performance in Cross-Country Skiing** *James E. Wolfe, Ed.D.*	15
Part II.	*Handicapped Sports*	25
Chapter 3.	**Fitness for the Handicapped: An Overview** *Robert C. Cantu, M.D.*	27
Chapter 4.	**A Study of Physiologic Parameters Before and After a Season of Wheelchair Basketball Competition** *Denis M. Desjardins, M.S.*	45
Chapter 5.	**Pulmonary and Cardiac Adjustments of Orthopedic Patients to a Mask-Flippers-Snorkel Aquatic Therapeutic Exercise Program** *Thomas G. Manfredi, Ph.D., Loretta DiPietro, M.S., and Michael Gavin, R.P.I., P.C.*	53
Chapter 6.	**Handicapped Skiing: An Overview** *David P. McCormick, M.D.*	63
Part III.	*Psychological Considerations*	71
Chapter 7.	**Behavior Coaching: Some Practical Aspects in the New Health Psychology** *Roger S. Zimmerman, Ph.D.*	73
Chapter 8.	**Using Perceived Exertion for the Prescription of Exercise in Healthy Adults** *Edmund J. Burke, Ph.D., and Marcia L. Collins, M.S.*	93

Part IV.   *Cardiopulmonary Considerations*   107

Chapter 9.   **Cardiopulmonary Exercise Testing:**
                  An Integrated Approach
                  Michael B. Zack, M.D.   109

Chapter 10.   **Basic Ventilatory Responses to Different**
                  Exercise Modalities
                  Timothy R. McConnell, Ph.D., David D. Swett,
                  Jr., M.D., Jose C. Missri, M.D., Robert M.
                  Jeresaty, M.D., and Arfan J. Al-Hani, M.D.   115

Chapter 11.   **Hypotension After Exercise and Relaxation**
                  Steven F. Siconolfi, Ph.D., Richard A.
                  Carleton, M.D., John P. Elder, Ph.D., and
                  Pamela A. Bouchard, M.S.N.   129

Chapter 12.   **Rehabilitation of the Pulmonary Patient**
                  Cynthia C. Zadai, M.S., R.P.T., and
                  Colleen M. Kigin, M.S., R.P.T.   139

Part V.   *Biomechanical Considerations*   161

Chapter 13.   **Power Output at Different Areas in the Range**
                  of Motion
                  John A. Clayton, Ph.D.   163

Chapter 14.   **Sculling: An Electromyographic Analysis**
                  Jonathan S. Herland, B.S.   169

Part VI.   *Team Sports Injury Prevention and*
                  Rehabilitation   177

Chapter 15.   **Injury Prevention and Rehabilitation in Baseball**
                  Robert C. Cantu, M.D.   179

Chapter 16.   **Injury Prevention and Rehabilitation in Track**
                  G. Richard Paul, M.D.   193

Chapter 17.   **Injuries in the Football Sports**
                  Lyle J. Micheli, M.D.   203

                  Index   211

Acknowledgments

This book contains selected papers presented at the Annual Meeting of the New England Chapter of the American College of Sports Medicine, November 19 and 20, 1982.

I would like to express sincere appreciation to the many contributing authors who forwarded their excellent manuscripts on schedule, thus enabling this effort to be timely. I also wish to thank Bernice McPhee, Director of Education and Training at Emerson Hospital and currently the Executive Secretary of the New England Chapter of the American College of Sports Medicine, who served as Annual Meeting Program Coordinator. Finally, a special word of thanks is extended to Pat Blackey for her skills in the preparation of this manuscript.

Robert C. Cantu, M.D.

Contributing Authors

Arfan J. Al-Hani, M.D.
Cardiac Rehabilitation Unit
Cardiology Section
Saint Francis Hospital and Medical Center
Hartford, Connecticut

Pamela Bouchard, M.S.N.
Division of Cardiology
Memorial Hospital
Pawtucket, Rhode Island

Edmund J. Burke, Ph. D.
Associate Professor of Physical Education
Springfield College
Springfield, Massachusetts

Robert C. Cantu, M.D.
Chief, Neurosurgical Service
Associate Chief, Department of Surgery
Director, Service of Sports Medicine
Emerson Hospital
Concord, Massachusetts

Richard A. Carleton, M.D.
Chief of Cardiology
Memorial Hospital
Pawtucket, Rhode Island

John A. Clayton, Ph.D.
Department of Physical Education
Northeastern University
Boston, Masschusetts

Marcia L. Collins, M.S.
Fitness Director
Green Mountain at Fox Run
Ludlow, Vermont

Denis M. Desjardins, M.S.
Bishop Hendricken High School
Warwick, Rhode Island

Loretta DiPietro, M.S.
Department of Public Health
Yale University
New Haven, Connecticut

John P. Elder, Ph.D.
Division of Cardiology
Memorial Hospital
Pawtucket, Rhode Island

Michael Gavin, R.P.T., P.C.
Chief Physical Therapist
Milford Hospital
Milford, Connecticut

Jonathan S. Herland, B.S.
Sargent College of Allied Health Professions
Boston University
Boston, Massachusetts

Robert M. Jeresaty, M.D.
Cardiac Rehabilitation Unit/Cardiology Section
Saint Francis Hospital and Medical Center
Hartford, Connecticut

Colleen M. Kigin, M.S., R.P.T.
Director, Chest Physical Therapy
Massachusetts General Hospital
Boston, Massachusetts

Thomas G. Manfredi, Ph.D.
Human Performance Laboratory
University of Rhode Island
Kingston, Rhode Island

Timothy R. McConnell, Ph.D.
Cardiac Rehabilitation Unit
Cardiology Section
Saint Francis Hospital and Medical Center
Hartford, Connecticut

David P. McCormick, M.D.
Pediatrician, Emerson Hospital
Concord, Massachusetts
Medical Staff, Children's Hospital Medical Center
Boston, Massachusetts

Lyle J. Micheli, M.D.
Department of Orthopedics
Harvard Medical School
Director, Division of Sports Medicine
Children's Hospital Medical Center
Boston, Massachusetts

José C. Missri, M.D.
Cardiac Rehabilitation Unit
Cardiology Section
Saint Francis Hospital and Medical Center
Hartford, Connecticut

G. Richard Paul, M.D.
Associate Professor of Orthopedics
Boston University School of Medicine
Director of Sports Medicine
Northeastern University
Team Surgeon, Boston Breakers
Boston, Massachusetts

Steven F. Siconolfi, Ph.D.
Director, Human Performance Laboratory
Division of Cardiology
Memorial Hospital
Pawtucket, Rhode Island

David D. Swett, Jr., M.D.
Cardiac Rehabilitation Unit
Cardiology Section
Saint Francis Hospital and Medical Center
Hartford, Connecticut

David G. Watson, M.B.B.S., M.R.C.P. (U.K.)
Pediatric Cardiologist
Emerson Hospital
Concord, Massachusetts

James E. Wolfe, Ed.D.
Professor of Physical Education
Dean Junior College
Franklin, Massachusetts

Michael B. Zack, M.D.
Clinical Assistant Professor of Medicine
Boston University School of Medicine
Boston, Massachusetts
Director of Pulmonary Medicine
Malden Hospital
Malden, Massachusetts

Cynthia C. Zadai, M.S., R.P.T.
Chief, Chest Physical Therapy
Beth Israel Hospital
Boston, Massachusetts

Roger S. Zimmerman, Ph.D.
Faculty, University of Southern Maine
Independent Practice
Portland, Maine

Predicting Sports Performance

1 Check Your Talent, Choose Your Sport

David G. Watson, M.B.B.S.

Currently, children of all ages are engaging in competitive and recreational sports in unprecedented numbers. Leagues for tennis, skiing, basketball, and skating are among the many competitive outlets available to today's growing athlete. Most children select a sport for their participation primarily because their peers accept it or because their parents have introduced it to them. Climate also can be influential in a child's selection of a sports activity. In California and Florida, for instance, tennis and swimming are favorites, whereas in the northern states, skiing and ice hockey are popular choices.

It is my opinion that many of these embryonic athletes are specializing too early. They do not fully explore the variety of sports and activities beyond those immediately available. In this chapter, ways in which children's athletic horizons may be broadened will be emphasized. One program for determining an individual's athletic talents requires that the young athlete complete a series of tests. A score is recorded for each test, and each score then is rated for the individual's age, sex, and stage of development. When all tests are completed, an overall profile of the child's athletic strengths and weaknesses emerges. The child's strengths can be compared with the skills and abilities needed for different sports, and his or her profile can be compared against that of established sports champions.

Such a profile can be helpful if the young athlete is interested in trying new sports. It can help the individual select sports in which he or she is more likely to succeed. However, this profile tests only for talent. It does not test for drive, ambition, or the will to win. A young competitor who lacks strong skills required for a certain sport still may be successful at that sport owing to a strong inner drive. Nonetheless, all these things being equal, the most talented athlete will be more successful.

Determination of Developmental Age

Before the tests can be employed, it is important to assess the young athlete's developmental age. At puberty, great leaps in strength and endurance are made and, as puberty develops at different ages for different children, it must be factored into an evaluation of the athletic profile. One method is to use the staging of Tanner and colleagues* in which pictures of breasts and genitals are compared with the individual child's physical build and a rating of pubertal development is made. This method has many drawbacks for large-scale use.

I have proposed an alternative assessment method called the *performance age*. The average girl begins puberty at approximately 10½ years of age, and the average boy at approximately 12 years of age. Since strength and endurance (performance) are more correlated with pubertal development than with chronologic age for many tests, the tests should be scored with developmental age rather than real age. There is a simple way to determine developmental age: Girls who have not started puberty use their real age until 10 years; from 10 until they first develop breasts ½ year is added for each year (e.g., a 12-year-old girl who has not developed breasts would have a performance age of 11). At the age when breasts develop, the girl's performance age is 10½. If she was 9 years old when this happened and she now is 12, her performance age is 10½ (at age 9) plus 3 (the number of years since puberty started), or 13½ years.

The same principle applies for boys. Thus, a 15-year-old boy who did not start puberty until 14 years of age would have a performance age of 12 (his performance age when puberty started) plus 1 (the number of years since puberty started), or 13 years. Puberty starts for boys when their penis and testicles begin to enlarge. They do not change much in size from birth until puberty.

Tests for Athletic Talent

The tests for athletic talent are divided into four groups: (1) muscle profile, (2) neurologic profile, (3) endurance, and (4) body composition profile. They are designed to be used by children with help from their friends or parents.

Muscle Profile

Performance age is used when scoring the group of tests composing the muscle profile. The muscles that move our arms, legs, and bodies are of two types—fast-contracting and slow-contracting. The fast-contracting muscles generate a lot of power quickly but tire easily. Slow-contracting muscles, on the other hand, achieve the same overall power as the fast-contracting muscles but do so slowly and efficiently. They go on contracting for much longer. They are called *endurance muscles*.

Test 1: Vertical Jump. The vertical jump (Table 1-1) tests for pure explosive power and measures one's fast-contracting muscles. The child

---
*J.M. Tanner, In Gardner, Lytt I., *Endocrine and Genetic Diseases of Childhood and Adolesence.* Philadelphia: W.B. Saunders, 1975, pp. 20-33.

Table 1-1
Test 1: Vertical Jump Performance Scores for Boys and Girls
of Various Ages

Performance Category	Score (in.) According to Performance Age				
	7–8 Yr.	9–10 Yr.	11–12 Yr.	13–14 Yr.	15–16 Yr.
Boys					
Good	11	12	13	20	22
Average	8	10	11	15	15
Poor	5	7	9	12	11
Girls					
Good	10	11	12	13	17
Average	7	9	10	11	12
Poor	4½	7	8	8	8½

should stand against a wall with chalk in his or her hand. The child makes a mark as high as possible on the wall, keeping his or her feet flat on the floor. Then the child jumps as high up the wall as possible and makes another mark high up. The difference between the marks is the measure of the vertical jump. This is repeated three times. Take the largest difference for the score.

Test 2: Fifty-Yard Sprint. A measured 50 yards, stopwatch, starter and a timer are needed for the 50-yard sprint. Several runs should be taken and the results should be averaged (Table 1-2). This test measures fast-contracting muscles and compares closely with the vertical jump.

Test 3: Chin-ups. For Test 3 (Table 1-3), a chin-up bar is gripped with the palms of one's hands facing oneself. The individual hangs with arms extended, then pulls up until his or her chin is above the bar. A return to the arms-extended position completes one chin-up. This should be repeated as

Table 1-2
Test 2: Fifty-Yard Sprint Performance Scores for Boys and Girls
of Various Ages

Performance Category	Score (sec.) According to Performance Age				
	9–10 Yr.	11–12 Yr.	13–14 Yr.	15–16 Yr.	17+ Yr.
Boys					
Good	7.5	7.1	6.5	6.2	6.0
Average	8.2	7.9	7.3	6.8	6.6
Poor	9.5	9.0	8.5	7.5	7.5
Girls					
Good	7.5	7.2	7.0	6.8	7.0
Average	8.6	8.1	7.9	7.8	7.9
Poor	9.9	9.4	9.8	8.8	9.0

Table 1-3
Test 3: Chin-ups Performance Scores for Boys and Girls of Various Ages

	Score (no.) According to Performance Age				
Performance Category	7–8 Yr.	9–10 Yr.	11–12 Yr.	13–14 Yr.	15–16 Yr.
Boys					
Good	5	10	10	10	14
Average	1½	3	3	4	6½
Poor	0	0	0	0	0
Girls					
Good	5	10	8	3	10
Average	1½	3	1	1	3
Poor	0	0	0	0	0

many times as possible. The test measures power-to-weight ratio or performance.

Neurologic Profile

One's real age is used in scoring the two tests in the neurologic profile, but adults use age 16.

Test 4: Hopscotch. On a pavement, a hopscotch course is marked in chalk as in Figure 1–1. Starting at A, the individual hops into each numbered square, turning at 9 and returning to A, and reversing the order for the return. After a trial run, completion of the course is timed with a stopwatch (Table 1–4). Left and right feet can be used simultaneously (e.g., the left foot in square 1 while the right foot is in square 2; then the right foot in square 3; followed by the left in square 4 while the right is in square 5, and so on). Each square should be touched in the correct order, but it is not necessary to keep one's feet inside the lines. This tests a person's agility, balance, and coordination.

Test 5: Ruler Drop. A 12-inch ruler is needed. While a friend holds the ruler vertically with the 0–inch mark at eye level, the person being tested places finger and thumb 1 inch apart at the zero-mark end of the ruler. Without warning, the friend should drop the ruler and the tested individual must

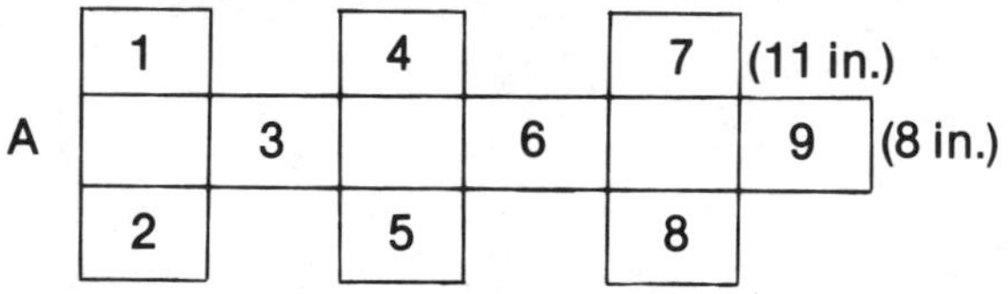

Figure 1–1. Hopscotch course for test 4 in the neurologic profile.

Table 1-4
Test 4: Hopscotch Performance Scores for Boys and Girls of Various Ages

Performance Category	Score (sec.) According to Chronologic Age				
	7–8 Yr.	9–10 Yr.	11–12 Yr.	13–14 Yr.	15–16 Yr.
Boys					
Good	6.0	4.5	4.2	4.4	4.4
Average	6.7	5.4	5.0	5.3	5.2
Poor	7.5	6.0	5.7	7.0	7.0
Girls					
Good	5.5	4.1	3.5	3.5	3.5
Average	6.2	4.8	3.9	4.0	4.7
Poor	7.5	6.5	5.2	5.4	5.5

catch the ruler and note where the top of the index finger is. This is repeated several times until three successive catches within ½ inch of one another are achieved (Table 1–5). This test measures one's reaction time. The quicker the reaction time, the shorter the distance the ruler drops before it is caught.

Endurance

Test 6: One-Mile Run. Performance age is used to score the endurance test (Table 1–6). A level measured mile and a watch with a sweep second hand are needed. A friend should pace the person being tested. A slow start should give way to a gradual increase in speed as the runner proceeds until the runner has some difficulty talking while running. The 1-mile running time measures one's endurance ability.

Body Composition Profile

In scoring the four tests that compose the body composition profile, performance age is used.

Table 1-5
Test 5: Ruler Drop Performance Scores for Boys and Girls of Various Ages

Performance Category	Score (in.) According to Chronologic Age				
	7–8 Yr.	9–10 Yr.	11–12 Yr.	13–14 Yr.	15–16 Yr.
Boys					
Good	8	5	4	5	5
Average	10	9.5	6.5	7.5	6
Poor	24	14	10	10	8
Girls					
Good	11	6	4	5	5
Average	18	10	7	6.5	6
Poor	24	14	10	10	8

Table 1-6
**Test 6: One-Mile Run Performance Scores for Boys and Girls
of Various Ages**

Performance Category	Score (min.) According to Performance Age				
	7–8 Yr.	9–10 Yr.	11–12 Yr.	13–14 Yr.	15–16 Yr.
Boys					
Good	8.2	7.0	6.5	6.7	5.7
Average	9.5	9.2	7.2	8.3	6.6
Poor	13.0	11.0	9.5	9.5	9.5
Girls					
Good	9.2	7.0	6.5	7.0	6.0
Average	11.3	11.0	7.0	8.3	7.0
Poor	14.0	12.0	9.5	9.7	9.5

Test 7: Height. Height (Table 1–7) and weight can be determined from standard growth charts. The ninetieth percentile is tall and the tenth percentile is short.

Test 8: Leg and Trunk Length. To determine one's leg and trunk length, one's height must be measured both while standing and while sitting. The standing height measurement is divided by the sitting height measurement, and the resulting ratio indicates how long one's limbs or legs are (Table 1–8). A ratio of 2 or more means long legs, whereas a ratio of 1.7 or less means a long trunk.

Test 9: Flexibility. Each of three flexibility subtests shown in Figure 1–2 are scored 1, 2, or 3. The total of these three scores will indicate overall flexibility: The higher the combined score is, the more flexible is the individual (Table 1–9).

Table 1-7
Test 7: Body Height of Boys and Girls of Various Ages

Height Category	Height (in.) According to Performance Age (yr)										
	7	8	9	10	11	12	13	14	15	16	17
Boys											
Tall	51	53	55	58	61	64	67	70	72	73	76
Average	48	50	52	54	56	59	62	64	66	68	70
Small	45	47	49	51	53	55	57	60	61	65	66
Girls											
Tall	51	54	56	59	62	64	66	68	68	68	69
Average	47	50	52	56	57	60	62	63	64	64	64
Small	44	47	49	51	53	56	58	60	60	61	61

Table 1-8
Test 8: Leg and Trunk Length as a Ratio of Standing Height to Sitting Height for Boys and Girls of Various Ages

| | *Ratios According to Performance Age (yr)* | | | | | | | | | | |
	7	*8*	*9*	*10*	*11*	*12*	*13*	*14*	*15*	*16*	*17*
Boys	1.83	1.86	1.89	1.89	1.93	1.94	1.96	1.96	1.94	1.94	1.93
Girls	1.87	1.88	1.9	1.92	1.93	1.94	1.92	1.92	1.91	1.91	1.90

Test 10: Lung Capacity. Into a 1-gallon plastic milk container the individual being tested should pour 1-pint increments of water, marking each pint level. The full bottle then is inverted under water. The person then takes a

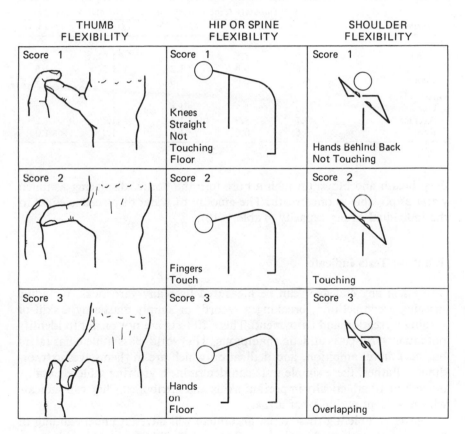

Figure 1-2. Three subtests for flexibility in the body composition profile.

Table 1-9
Test 9: Flexibility Performance Scores for Boys and Girls of Various Ages

	Average Combined Score from Three Flexibility Subtests[a] According to Performance Age			
	9–10 Yr.	11–12 Yr.	13–14 Yr.	15–16 Yr.
Boys	6	6	5.5	5.0
Girls	6	5.6	6.7	7

[a]See Figure 1-2.

Table 1-10
Test 10: Lung Capacity Determined by Water Displacement for Boys and Girls of Various Ages

Performance Category	Lung Capacity (pints) According to Performance Age (yr)				
	7–8 Yr.	9–10 Yr.	11–12 Yr.	13–14 Yr.	15–16 Yr.
Boys					
Good	1.0	1.5	1.5	1.9	2.2
Average	0.6	0.8	1.2	1.3	1.6
Poor	0.5	0.6	1.0	1.0	1.1
Girls					
Good	1.0	1.2	1.6	1.7	1.8
Average	0.7	1.0	1.3	1.3	1.2
Poor	0.6	0.6	1.0	1.0	1.0

deep breath and blows through a hose into the bottle, displacing as much water as possible in one breath. The amount of water displaced is equal to the individual's lung capacity (Table 1–10).

What the Tests Indicate

Success in any endeavor can be measured by many yardsticks, including winning a competition, breaking a record, or simply mastering a skill or finding recreation and enjoyment. These 10 tests are not meant to identify potential world-class athletic champions. The world-class athlete has talent but also drive, ambition, and dedication which are in themselves extraordinary. Rather, these simple tests can determine a growing athlete's ability in each of 10 athletically important skills and attributes. They can indicate who has talent and in what areas.

After completing these tests, an athlete will have an understanding of his or her strengths and weaknesses. He or she will learn why his or her performance in one sport far surpasses performance in another. The athlete may discover that he or she has potential for sports activities not yet tried. He or she will see what natural weakness can be improved. These tests are designed to help the athlete understand better his or her capabilities. For younger people, they can serve as a guide in choosing sports best suited to an individual's abilities. The following are some examples of using these tests to profile successful athletes:

A downhill skier has a good vertical jump score and is agile (does well on test 4).

A cross-country skier will do well in the 1-mile run.

Baseball requires agility (test 4), quick reflexes (test 5), and fast muscles (tests 1 and 2).

Gymnasts are agile (test 4) and have a good power-to-weight ratio (test 3).

Swimmers have long trunks (test 8) and are flexible (test 9).

Scoring the Tests

A person's talent is scored by comparing his or her results with the tables provided for each test. Adults should use 16 years in scoring, but children and adolescents should determine their score using their real age or their performance age, according to the test specifications. Tables 1 through 10 are mostly a tabulation of results from test scores by children and adolescents, age 7 to 17 years, who were randomly selected from the physical education classes at elementary, middle, and high schools in Westford, Massachusetts.

The person being tested should make a note of the tests in which he or she excels. Of course, not all the tests are ability tests: In some, such as those for height and body composition, one size or shape might suit one sport whereas another size or shape is better in a different sport (e.g., tall for basketball but small for gymnastics). Once the tests have been scored and the individual's strengths have been identified by high scores in particular tests, that person's talent for certain sports activities can be determined.

Finding One's Talent

By grouping sports according to similar talent requirements, a profile is created that can be matched with an individual's results.

Team Field Sports

As he cuts left, dodges right, then accelerates past a diving defender, Tony Dorsett demonstrates talents needed for field and ball control sports, such as American football, soccer, field hockey, and rugby; lacrosse, ice hockey, and basketball are others. His quickness comes from fast twitch muscle fibers. He performs well in the vertical jump. Body control and timing are important, and a good score in the hopscotch test demonstrates this.

Additional talents are helpful in some sports. For example, soccer players are much smaller and demonstrate more endurance ability than football players. Trunk ratio (a low number for a low center of gravity) is important for participation in ice hockey or to succeed in the position of a football lineman. Endurance is crucial in field hockey as well as soccer. A person of small size is more likely to succeed in soccer, whereas a larger person is better suited to football. Quick reflexes (indicated by a high score in the ruler drop) are needed by goalies. Someone who is tall and has long arms is potentially well suited to basketball. A simple test to determine whether one's arms are long is to have a friend measure from fingertip to fingertip of one's outstretched arms. If this measurement is equal to or greater than one's height measurement, the arms are considered to be long.

Bat and Racquet Sports

It is match point, and Martina Navratilova looms over the net. Her opponent rifles a low return. Navratilova's lightning movement and a steel wrist angle the ball for the winning point. Tennis is one of many bat and racquet sports, including baseball, cricket, squash, racquetball, paddle tennis, and pelota, which require quick reaction, rapid last-minute adjustments, and fast muscles. A good score on both the ruler drop and vertical jump tests will indicate potentially successful athletes in these sports. Taller-than-average people who demonstrate these abilities may be especially well suited to the position of a baseball pitcher or cricket bowler.

Dance Sports

Gliding across the ice, Dorothy Hamill jumps and spins with the grace and beauty of a gazelle in flight. She is literally one in a million. Her effortless performance is deceiving. Special skills and thousands of hours of practice are the essential components of her success.

Figure skating represents the dance sports, which also include ballet, gymnastics, diving, and downhill and freestyle skiing. To do well in these sports, small size, quick muscles (the vertical jump), good body control (the hopscotch test), flexibility (test 9), and a good power-to-weight ratio (chin-ups) are helpful.

Swimming

Standing on the starting block, Mark Spitz is not notably distinguishable from the many fine athletes with whom he competes. He is tall and slim with large hands. In the water, though, he surges to the front on the way to yet another gold medal. In addition to numerous hours of hard training, a long trunk, large lung capacity, and flexibility (especially at the shoulder) contribute to one's potential success in this sport.

A low standing height–to–sitting height ratio is indicative of a long trunk. Flexibility can be demonstrated by a high score on test 9. Sprint swimmers should perform well in the vertical jump and chin-ups tests, in contrast to endurance swimmers, who should perform well in the 1-mile run but who will do poorly in the vertical jump and chin-ups tests.

Track and Field Sports

Bruce Jenner, winner of the 1976 Olympic gold medal for the Decathlon, does not represent an enigma in modern international sports. There is no such person as an all-round athlete. Rather, Jenner has the physique to do very well in most track and field sports; he has the fast muscles for all the sports, is flexible for hurdles, and has a strong flexible upper body for the throwing and pole vault events. In addition, he has trained enough for endurance to perform respectably in the 1-mile run.

All track and field sports except distance running require fast or explosive muscles. Even the 1-mile run requires sprinting ability. It is the endurance events in which decathletes perform poorly. Running distances of more than 1 mile, like most other endurance sports, requires smaller body size and strong endurance muscles. The true endurance athlete is completely opposite from the sprinter. No one can do both well. The good sprinter is, by necessity, a poor distance runner. The staying power of endurance athletes can be attributed to their muscles' efficient use of energy. As in a high-mileage car, efficiency and acceleration do not go together.

A 3-mile run would be the best test for endurance, but currently available data allow us to use only the 1-mile run. This test can be applied to potential runners, swimmers, cross-country skiers, and bicycle racers. Long legs also are helpful to endurance athletes. The sprint sports (including the 50- to 800-m run, the long jump, triple jump, and high jump, and throwing events such as the pole vault) all require a good vertical jump score. Hurdles require flexibility. Throwing events, including the pole vault, also require upper body strength, flexibility, and coordination. Long legs (a high center of gravity) are needed for the high jump.

2 Anthropometric, Physiologic, and Psychological Measures to Predict Performance in Cross-Country Skiing

James E. Wolfe, Ed.D.

Cross-country skiing is a well-established winter adventure activity that is both challenging and stressful. Often called *ski touring* or *nordic skiing*, it is a fast-growing sport, an alternative to jogging that people can enjoy on a snow-covered golf course or in deep birch or pine forests. In recent years, there has developed a need for cross-country skiing competition which is based primarily on the American public's growing interest in cross-country skiing. The United States Ski Association (USSA) holds a total of 200 national citizens' cross-country skiing competitions in nine regional divisions. As a skier progresses from casual recreational outings to competitive citizens' races, the physiologic and skill requirements greatly increase. An assessment of the requirements of cross-country skiing performance is needed to evaluate the demands on the body during competitive racing.

The studies I reviewed in preparing the present study described in this chapter indicate that body composition and physical work capacity influence an individual's ability to perform in an athletic event. The psychology of sport performance has also received considerable emphasis in the literature, especially with regard to anxiety and sport competition. Early investigations of oxygen requirements for cross-country skiing and endurance-related sports included studies by Astrand [1], Saltin [2], and Hanson and Tabakin [3]. The testing of the U.S. National Nordic Ski Team members originated with Dr. Marvin Clein of the University of Denver and Dr. Arthur Dickinson of the University of Colorado: Physiologic and psychological tests were given to collect knowledge about athletes to use in increasing their levels of performance [4]. More recent studies by Hanson [5, 6], Sinning et al. [7], Ruhling and Storer [8], and Haymes et al. [9] have dealt with physical training, body composition, and oxygen intake requirements for cross-country ski racers. A variety of tests have been used to measure anxiety to predict performance during stress and competition [10]. After reviewing these various predictors of anxiety, I selected for use in this study the Illinois Sport Competition Anxiety Test (SCAT) developed by Martens [11] because of its reliability for prediction of the precompetition anxiety state. The importance of anthropometric,

15

physiologic, and psychological variables for success in the sport of cross-country skiing resulted in test selection to assess these areas [12].

The Study

The purpose of this study was to determine if the selected variables of lean body weight, physical work capacity, and precompetition anxiety were related to the successful performance of cross-country skiers in competitive racing. Other independent variables included the subject's age, height, and total body weight.

Procedure for Collecting Data

Subjects. Thirty-five men and forty women between the ages of 14 and 53 years who were nonclassified or class C* cross-country ski racing competitors volunteered to serve as subjects. The mean age and standard deviation values for the men and women were 17.0 ± 3.8, and 22.29 ± 5.2 respectively. All subjects participated in ski training camps and cross-country ski races sponsored by the Eastern Division of the USSA. These training camps were held at three nordic ski areas: Craftsbury Ski Academy, Vermont, (group 1) hosted 27 female participants; Williams College Ski Area, Massachusetts, (group 2) hosted 14 male subjects; and Bretton Woods Ski Area, New Hampshire, hosted 21 men (group 3A) and 13 women (group 3B).

Test Selection and Administration. Direct methods for measuring physical work capacity (PWC) and lean body weight (LBW) using complex and precise laboratory equipment were not applicable for use in cross-country ski training camps. Therefore, skin-fold measurements were used to determine LBW, a submaximal step test was used to determine PWC, and SCAT was used to measure precompetition anxiety.

Skin-fold measurements were taken using the Lange skin-fold calipers (Lange Calipers Mfg., Cambridge, Md.). In men, abdominal and thigh skin-folds were measured. In women, the suprailiac and thigh areas were measured. Equations established by Wilmore and Behnke [13] and Pollock et al. [14] (reliability 0.80 and 0.78) were used in determining body density. The percent of body fat was calculated using a formula developed by Siri [15].

A submaximal ergometer step test developed by the International Committee for the Standardization of Physical Fitness Tests was used to predict

---

*Ski racers who have fewer than eighty points in competition classification by the United States Ski Association are considered class C competitors. Nonclassified skiers are those with no competition experience in USSA sanctioned races.

maximal oxygen intake ($\dot{V}o_2$ max) and determine PWC. The step test used a platform with step levels 10, 20, 30, 40, and 50 cm high. The subject stepped onto and down from the step ergometer for 3 minutes at a rate of 30 steps per minute at each of the specified step levels. Heart rate was monitored by a portable heart rate monitor (Parks & Co. model 503; Parks Electronic Laboratories, Beauerton, Ore.). The test ended when the heart rate of the subject reached a level of approximately 80 percent of the maximum value for his or her age group (e.g., 156 beats per minute for people aged 21 to 35 years) [14].

The Illinois SCAT questionnaire was administered to subjects just prior to their competing in a cross-country ski race.

Each subject's skiing performance was evaluated by recording the time he or she required to complete the cross-country ski race.

Results

The t tests to compare the group means for all six independent variables revealed significant differences, indicating that the four groups represented different populations and, therefore, they were handled separately in statistical analysis (Tables 2–1 through 2–3).

Intercorrelations were computed between the previous six independent variables and the dependent variable of ski race time for the four groups (Tables 2–4 through 2–7). The demographic variables of age, height, and weight did not appear to influence ski racing performance. Intercorrelations indicated significant relationships between percent of body fat and ski race time in one group (Table 2–6), negative relationships between $\dot{V}o_2$ max and

Table 2–1
Means, Standard Deviations (SD), and t Ratios
for Independent Variable Values for Men

Independent Variable	Group 2: Williams College (n = 14)		Group 3A: Bretton Woods (n = 21)		Difference	t
	Mean	SD	Mean	SD		
Body fat (%)	10.26	1.10	11.44	2.04	1.18	1.97
$\dot{V}o_2$ max (ml/kg/min)	33.28	4.39	36.34	4.40	3.06	2.01
SCAT	25.36	2.94	21.86	4.48	3.5	2.57[a]
Age (yr)	15.14	.74	21.04	10.51	5.9	4.18[a]
Height (cm)	171.08	7.47	180.52	5.35	9.44	4.35[a]
Weight (kg)	56.06	7.07	75.75	6.06	19.69	8.80[a]

[a]t = 2.04 necessary for significance at 0.05 level.
SCAT = Illinois Sport Competition Anxiety Test.

Table 2–2
Means, Standard Deviations (SD), and t Ratios
for Independent Variable Values for Women

Independent Variable	Group 1: Craftsbury ($n = 27$)		Group 3B: Bretton Woods ($n = 13$)		Difference	t
	Mean	SD	Mean	SD		
Body fat (%)	15.79	1.85	15.68	2.31	0.11	0.162
$\dot{V}o_2$ max (ml/kg/min)	33.19	4.70	33.51	4.34	0.32	0.041
SCAT	22.89	4.48	23.54	4.18	0.65	0.439
Age (yr)	15.85	1.0	19.38	5.91	3.53	2.95[a]
Height (cm)	163.75	5.80	163.49	6.52	0.26	0.15
Weight (kg)	54.49	5.08	51.5	4.62	2.99	1.80

[a] $t = 2.02$ necessary for significance at 0.05 level.
SCAT = Sport Competition Anxiety Test.

Table 2–3
Means, Standard Deviations (SD), and t Ratios
for Independent Variables for Men and Women

Independent Variable	Groups 1 and 3B: ($n = 40$)		Groups 2 and 3A: ($n = 35$)		Difference	t
	Mean	SD	Mean	SD		
Body fat (%)	15.76	2.01	10.97	1.82	4.79	10.75[a]
$\dot{V}o_2$ max (ml/kg/min)	33.29	4.59	35.12	4.65	1.83	1.71
SCAT	23.10	4.40	23.26	4.29	0.16	0.15
Age (yr)	17.0	3.85	22.29	10.06	5.29	3.04[a]
Height (cm)	163.67	6.06	176.75	7.82	13.08	8.04[a]
Weight (kg)	55.46	5.13	67.88	11.62	12.42	1.40

[a] $t = 2.00$ necessary for significance at 0.05 level.
SCAT = Sport Competition Anxiety Test.

Table 2–4
Correlation Matrix of Craftsbury Ski Academy
(Group 1) Data ($n = 27$)

Variable	1	2	3	4	5	6	7
Age (yr)		0.2645	0.2679	−0.0957	0.3553	0.1112	0.1741
Height (cm)			0.7451[a]	0.1816	0.0476	−0.1290	0.0024
Weight (kg)				0.0594	0.1814	0.0524	0.1940
$\dot{V}o_2$ max (ml/kg/min)					−0.0121	−0.0515	−0.2469
Body fat (%)						0.1505	0.2753
SCAT (score)							−0.0175
3.5-km race (min:sec)							

[a] .05 level.
SCAT = Sport Competition Anxiety Test.

Table 2–5
Correlation Matrix of Williams College Ski Area
(Group 2) Data ($n = 14$)

Variable	1	2	3	4	5	6	7
Age (yr)		0.3042	0.2241	−0.1659	0.0328	−0.2522	−0.0116
Height (cm)			0.8019[a]	0.2092	−0.0124	0.0602	0.1483
Weight (kg)				0.3642	−0.0396	0.1252	−0.0833
V̇o$_2$ max (ml/kg/min)					−0.0434	−0.1191	−0.7034[a]
Body fat (%)						0.2183	0.1937
SCAT (score)							0.0516
3.5-km race (min:sec)							

[a] .05 level.
SCAT = Sport Competition Anxiety Test.

Table 2–6
Correlation Matrix of Bretton Woods Ski Area
(Group 3A) Data ($n = 21$)

Variable	1	2	3	4	5	6	7
Age (yr)		0.1816	0.2323	0.0977	−0.0848	0.1230	0.0545
Height (cm)			0.5854[a]	−0.1857	0.0241	0.0332	0.1226
Weight (kg)				−0.4066	0.5921[a]	−0.0327	0.3118
V̇o$_2$ max (ml/kg/min)					−0.5417[a]	−0.0477	−0.4921[a]
Body fat (%)						−0.0259	0.5615[a]
SCAT (score)							0.2874
10.3-km race (min:sec)							

[a] .05 level.
SCAT = Sport Competition Anxiety Test.

Table 2–7
Correlation Matrix of Bretton Woods Ski Area
(Group 3B) Data ($n = 13$)

Variable	1	2	3	4	5	6	7
Age (yr)		0.1782	−0.0193	0.5632[a]	−0.5431	0.4083	0.1560
Height (cm)			0.2063	0.2412	−0.1499	−0.0519	−0.1707
Weight (kg)				−0.0266	0.4153	−0.1070	−0.4030
V̇o$_2$ max (ml/kg/min)					−0.4230	0.2449	−0.2528
Body fat (%)						−0.1947	−0.3333
SCAT (score)							0.2840
10.3-km race (min:sec)							

[a] .05 level.
SCAT = Sport Competition Anxiety Test.

ski race time in two groups (Tables 2-5, 2-6), and low correlations between SCAT and ski race time in all groups.

The cumulative effects of two variables (LBW and $\dot{V}o_2$ max in two of the group studies) and ski race time yielded significant multiple correlations in three of the groups (groups 2, 3A, and 3B). When three variables—LBW, $\dot{V}o_2$ max, and SCAT—were used, significant correlations were found in the same three groups (Table 2-8).

The correlation values obtained for the multiple regression equations were significant beyond the 0.05 level for the use of LBW, PWC, and SCAT test raw scores to predict ski race time (Table 2-9). This finding confirmed

Table 2-8
Correlation Between Two or More Prediction Variables and Ski Race Time

Group	Prediction Variables	R	R^2
1	% Body fat and $\dot{V}o_2$ max	0.3675	0.1350
	% Body fat, Vo_2 max, and SCAT	0.3745	0.1402
2	Vo_2 max and % body fat	0.7222[a]	0.5216
	Vo_2 max, % body fat, and SCAT	0.7293[a]	0.5319
3A	% Body fat and SCAT	0.6375[a]	0.4064
	% Body fat, SCAT, and $\dot{V}o_2$ max	0.6688[a]	0.4473
3B	% Body fat and $\dot{V}o_2$ max	0.5481[a]	0.3004
	% Body fat, $\dot{V}o_2$ max, and SCAT	0.6288[a]	0.3954

[a] .05 level.
SCAT = Sport Competition Anxiety Test.

Table 2-9
Equations to Predict Final Ski Race Time (Rt) from Prediction Variables of Lean Body Weight (LBW), Physical Work Capacity (PWC), and Sport Competition Anxiety Test (SCAT)

Group	Equations	R	R^2	Standard Error
1	Rt = 0.2751(LBW) + 9.4637	0.2751	0.0757	1.6990
	Rt = 0.2721(LBW) − 0.2437($\dot{V}o_2$) + 12.4346	0.3675	0.1350	1.6775
2	Rt = −0.70346($\dot{V}o_2$) + 20.5389	0.7035[a]	0.4949	1.3336
3A	Rt = 0.5615(LBW) + 11.0029	0.5615[a]	0.3153	10.0756
	Rt = 0.5693(LBW) + 0.3021(SCAT) − 6.5917	0.6375[a]	0.4064	9.6379
	Rt = 0.4382(LBW) + 0.2872(SCAT − 0.2412 ($\dot{V}o_2$) + 25.8088	0.6688[a]	0.4473	9.5699
3B	Rt = −0.3334(LBW) + 56.1757	0.3334	0.1112	3.9919
	Rt = −0.5365(LBW) − 0.4801($\dot{V}o_2$) + 75.9812	0.5481[a]	0.3004	3.7144
	Rt = −0.5011(LBW) − 0.5434($\dot{V}o_2$) + 0.3195 (SCAT) + 69.9379	0.6288[a]	0.3954	3.6400

[a] .05 level.

that the three tests contained high predictive validity of the cross-country ski racer's performance.

Discussion

A major objective of this study was to determine the influence of LBW, PWC, and SCAT on the performance of recreational citizens' racers in cross-country skiing. The subjects of this study are classified a grade below the more experienced intercollegiate and national-level skiers that were reported in the literature. These experienced performers recorded extremely high values for $\dot{V}o_2$ max and had a low percentage of lean body fat. Studies reported by Saltin and Astrand [2], Hanson [5, 6], Sinning et al. [7], Ruhling and Storer [8], and Berg et al. [17] reveal the physiologic characteristic of national and elite performances. The study of intercollegiate skiers by Niinimaa et al. [18] reveals somewhat lower values of $\dot{V}o_2$ max and LBW for this level of competition (Table 2–10).

The psychological aspects of cross-country ski racing have not been studied except for some limited reports on the U.S. National Nordic Ski Team [4]. The recreational citizens' racer has had limited experience in competitive racing and, therefore, cannot be compared with the experienced or elite national competitor. The results of this study indicate that precompetition state anxiety was not a factor in determining performance for the citizens' racer.

Table 2–10
Body Composition and $\dot{V}o_2$ max of Cross-Country Skiers Reported in Selected Studies

Study[a]	Performance Level	n	Sex	Body Fat (%)	$\dot{V}o_2$ max (ml/kg/min) Mean	Highest
Saltin and Astrand, 1967 [2]	Swedish National	5	M		83.0	85.0
Hanson, 1973 [5]	U.S. Nordic	7	M	7.4–10.1	75.0	88.3
Sinning et al., 1975 [7]	U.S. Nordic	11	M	7.2		
		5	F	16.1		
Hanson, 1975 [6]	U.S. Nordic	7	M	12.0	64.6[b]	
		2	F	16.7	64.6[b]	
Berg et al., 1978 [17]	Swedish		M		82.0[b]	94.0
	National	11[c]	F		82.0[b]	77.0
Ruhling and Storer, 1978 [8]	College	1	M	13.9		76
Niinimaa et al., 1978 [18]	College	10	M	12.5	63.9	70.6
Wolfe (present study)	Citizens'	35	M	10.97	35.11	43.5
	racers	40	F	15.76	33.29	43.6

[a]Refer to related literature.
[b]Combined mean score.
[c]Only total group number available.

The physiologic variables indicated to be important by studies of superior cross-country performers are evident in the recreational racer. The effects realized through training as documented by Hanson [6], Ruhling and Storer [8], and others are no different for the previously untrained skiers who are undergoing physical training, polishing their skiing techniques, and making psychological preparations for the upcoming winter season. It is postulated, therefore, that increased work capacity (PWC) through progressive accomplishment of a given work measurement should be of assistance to a racer's success. As Hanson [5, 6] has previously stated in discussing the U.S. National Nordic Team, "The physiological and psychological variables cannot be relied upon as total prediction of racing success; other neuromuscular factors such as coordination and strength, as well as skiing technique play an important role in competitive success" [7]. It was the intent of this study to learn more concerning the physiologic and psychological demands of cross-country skiing at the recreational citizens' race level. Recommendations for future studies would include assessment of training practice competition anxiety and additional methods to determine body composition and maximal oxygen intake, possibly in a controlled laboratory environment.

References

1. Astrand, P.-O., Saltin, B.   Maximal oxygen uptake and heart rate in various types of muscular activity. *J. Appl. Physiol.* 16:977, 1961.

2. Saltin, B., Astrand, P.-O.   Maximal oxygen uptake in athletes. *J. Appl. Physiol.* 23(3):353–358, 1967.

3. Hanson, J.S., Tabakin, B.   Electromyographic telemetry in skiers: anticipatory and recovery rate during competition. *N. Engl. J. Med.* 271(4):181–185, 1964.

4. Cross, L.   Skier performance measured. *Ski Racing* 6:5, 1973.

5. Hanson, J.S.   Maximal exercise performance in members of the U.S. Nordic Ski Team. *J. Appl. Physiol.* 35(5):592–595, 1973.

6. Hanson, J.S.   Decline of physiologic training effects during the competitive season in members of the U.S. Nordic Ski Team. *Med. Sci. Sports* 7(3):213–216, 1975.

7. Sinning, W.E., Cunningham, L.N., Racaniello, A.P., Sholes, J.L.   Body composition and somatotype of male and female nordic skiers. *Res. Q.* 48(4):741, 1977.

8. Ruhling, R.O., Storer, T.W.   Physiological Response to On-Snow Cross-Country Ski Training. Presented at the International Congress of Sports Sciences, University of Alberta, July 1978.

9. Haymes, E.M., Dickinson, A.L., Sparks, K.O. Physiological Characteristics of Champion Skiers. Paper presented at the American Alliance for Health, Physical Education, and Recreation Convention, Kansas City, Missouri, April 8, 1978.

10. Klauora, P. Application of the Spielberger Trait State Anxiety Model and STAI in Precompetition Research. Ph.D. diss., University of Alberta, 1974.

11. Martens, R. *Sport Competition Anxiety Test.* Champaign, Ill.: Human Kinetics Publishers, 1977.

12. Martens, R., Simon, J.A. Comparison of three predictors of state anxiety when competing. *Res. Q.* 47(3):381–387, 1976.

13. Wilmore, J.H., Behnke, A.R. An anthropometric estimation of body's density and lean body weight in young men. *J. Appl. Physiol.* 27:25–31, 1969.

14. Pollock, M.L., et al. Prediction of Body Density in Young Men and Middle-Aged Women. Paper presented at the annual meeting of the American College of Sports Medicine, 1974.

15. Siri, W.E. Body Composition from Fluid Spaces and Density. Donner Laboratory. Medical Physics Report 19. Berkeley: University of California, 1956.

16. Larson, L.A. *Fitness, Health and Work Capacity.* New York: Macmillan Publishing, 1974.

17. Berg, U., Thorstensson, A., Sjodin, B., et al. Maximal oxygen uptake and muscle fiber types in trained and untrained humans. *Med. Sci. Sports* 10(3):151–154, 1978.

18. Niinimaa, V., Dyon, M., Shephard, R.J. Performance and efficiency of intercollegiate cross-country skiers. *Med. Sci. Sports* 10(2):91–93, 1978.

II Handicapped Sports

3 Fitness for the Handicapped: An Overview

Robert C. Cantu, M.D.

Physical handicaps include hereditary (congenital) birth defects, all in utero birth defects, and the acquired loss of a portion of the body, either anatomically (by amputation) or functionally (by neurologic impairment). For most individuals, recreation provides a pleasurable and purposeful means of using leisure time. For the severely disabled—especially those who, because they cannot work or find employment, may have entire lives of leisure—recreation may assume a far more significant role. For many handicapped people, recreational activities will be the sole means of their interaction in the world at large, integrating them into society.

Sports activity, in addition to providing important social contact, may also provide the opportunity to improve muscular function in a particular disability, thus complementing whatever physiotherapy may be in progress. Recreational activities may even accomplish specific functional treatment objectives not attainable with other therapeutic media. Physical motions not possible through various occupational therapy crafts have been witnessed during games. Most important is the keen interest and spirit that sports and games generate, increasing motivation, physical tolerance, and self-confidence, because emphasis is shifted away from the disability to the activity.

Recreational activity also may provide a sense of freedom otherwise unknown to the disabled. Consider the different perspective an otherwise wheelchair-bound paraplegic has from the saddle of a horse or the seat of a kayak shooting the rapids, or from a sailplane soaring high above the earth. The emotional benefits of exercise, including aesthetic enjoyment, opportunity for personal expression, and enriching life experiences, are even greater than the physical benefits for the physically handicapped. The therapeutic benefits are obvious.

Historical Perspectives

Humankind's genuine concern for and systematic efforts to aid the handicapped date back approximately 200 years. One of the early leaders whose philosophic and educational writings provided spiritual impetus was the Swiss-French philosopher Jean Jacques Rousseau. For the first hundred of

27

those 200 years, essentially all the pioneers in work for the handicapped were European. French leaders included Jean Itard, Eduard Sequin, and Alfred Binet, whose research was on the mentally handicapped. Sign language for the deaf was developed by Abbe Sicard, and writing for the blind by Louis Braille. Johann Pestalozzi was a leader in Switzerland, Maria Montessori in Rome, and Alfred Adler and Agust Aickhorn in Austria.

In the last half century, the United States has become the leader in many aspects of research, services, and progress for children and adults with physical, mental, and emotional disabilities. The economic resources that provide freedom of investigation in the United States have afforded a climate for unsurpassed growth of theory, research, experimentation, and demonstration projects. Since World War II, especially, there also has been a notable improvement in public attitudes toward the disabled. This has resulted in new legislation, funding, institutions, and many novel approaches toward treatment of the handicapped.

Physiology of Exercise for the Disabled

It has been shown that the physically handicapped can achieve the same physical and emotional benefits from exercise as do those of us who are not disabled. In one study, the fitness test results of a group of wheelchair athletes were compared with those of nonwheelchair athletes. The same increased aerobic capacity and overall training effect was seen for arm exercising as has been shown for leg exercising (as in runners). The wheelchair athletes had significantly higher oxygen uptakes and lower resting and exertional heart rates. Other studies have shown the increased blood flow in regularly exercised arms as compared with those not so physically trained.

Selection of a Recreational Pursuit

Special Considerations in Individual Choice

Able-bodied individuals have varied personalities, temperaments, and physical characteristics that result in different recreational preferences. The presence of physical disability does not change these inherent traits. Although most handicapped people can participate in most recreational pursuits with special equipment, certain factors must be considered in the selection of an activity for each individual. First, it is important that the particular physical activity selected for participation by the handicapped individual provide him or her with an opportunity for enjoyment and success while not being potentially dangerous because of his or her specific disability.

Second, there will be differing needs and experiences associated with, and differing implications of, the particular medical affliction. For example, the requirements and approach to activity for the congenital paraplegic from a myelomeningocele, the paraplegic from an athletic injury, and the paraplegic from terminal cancer, multiple sclerosis, or some other progressive disease are vastly different. People recovering from an injury or illness must be guided toward activities that require progressively increased physical strength and endurance, whereas those afflicted with relentlessly progressive illness should become involved in activities that they can pursue regardless of diminishing physical activity.

The choice of an activity also must reflect the tastes of the individual, the type and degree of his or her handicap, and, to a large extent, his or her determination and motivation. A flexible approach is required for each person, especially when multiple handicaps, coordination problems, and strength deficits are present. In addition, the variation in duration of the handicaps and natural course of the affliction must be taken into account.

Money, too, must be considered, since many disabled people are not well off financially and some sports are expensive. However, I believe that the disabled should never adopt the attitude that cost will prevent their participation in a sport. Given adequate determination and motivation, financial barriers can be overcome; there are many ways that money can be raised for special equipment, courses, and the like.

The Variety of Sports Activities from which the Disabled May Choose

What makes many athletic pursuits possible is special physical equipment. The key to skiing for the amputee, for instance, is the outrigger. This is a ski tip attached by a hinged mount to an adjustable metal crutch. Amputee skiers use two outriggers in a manner similar to using a crutch, except that when skiing they lean forward on the outriggers for balance. Some outriggers are fitted with a spring-loaded spike that plunges several inches into the snow from the center of the ski. This acts much like a conventional ski pole to afford assistance on the level or uphill grades. With practice and conditioning, some users of the outriggers have achieved amazing performances on even the most difficult slalom courses.

The unilateral leg amputee who is otherwise in good condition often finds slalom waterskiing very easy to master. Here, only the standard ski is used and no special equipment is required. Leaning forward over the ski before the boat accelerates aids in reducing the force on the one leg at the start. Once the boat accelerates, the amputee in this position in essence body-planes to the upright position and then stands on the one leg. The increased surface area of the amputee's chest aids in bringing the ski on top of the water more quickly. Waterskiing can also be enjoyed by the blind and by arm amputees.

There seems to be no limit to the activities in which amputees can engage. With careful planning, the lower-extremity amputee can even sky dive and withstand the impact on landing. Just as some of our spacecrafts parachute into the ocean, the amputee sky diver can find a soft landing in a lake, reservoir, or similar body of water. Just as the Russians use the desert for landing their spacecrafts, so, too, a sandpit can serve as an alternative landing site for skydiving amputees.

Paraplegics and bilateral lower-extremity amputees have taken up a variety of hazardous activities, including mountain climbing, repelling down sheer mountain cliffs, and parakiting behind a speeding car. Scuba diving presents no problem when a special shortened wet suit with flippers firmly attached to the suit just below the stumps is worn. Sailing, sledding, canoeing, angling, rock climbing, cave exploring, and hang gliding have been done.

Horseback riding can be enjoyed by the bilateral amputee with or without prostheses, using a safety belt similar to those in automobiles to hold the amputee in the saddle. Horseback riding also is a favorite activity of many people who suffer from mental illness, cerebral palsy, or congenital, hereditary, neurologic, and traumatic conditions, and of the blind, the deaf, and the limbless. Although some may not progress beyond walking on a horse, others will acquire new skills and freedom and be able to join leisure activities on a par with able-bodied riders. Regardless of the level of skill acquired, all experience a feeling of independence. While riding, they can largely forget their disability and, regardless of the terrain, go wherever they want. The sights, sounds, smells, and sensations of being outdoors provide immense enjoyment. Aside from being an aerobic exercise, horseback riding allows for improvement of one's balance, coordination, and agility, heightens body awareness, and provides for relaxation and stretching of tight structures. An element of danger also is present, which normally is absent from the lives of most disabled people and which they generally find very stimulating.

Today, riding therapy has assumed a major role in the treatment of children with physical, emotional, and intellectual handicaps. Elsebet Bodtker of Norway, a trained physiotherapist, is a famed pioneer in this field. Recognizing the unique therapeutic values of horseback riding, both in developing physical skills and in encouraging self-confidence, she started the world's first riding school for disabled children in 1953. Twenty years later in 1973, the school hosted a world conference on riding therapy. Only very recently has the United States acknowledged riding therapy with wide acceptance. However, the Cheff Center for the Handicapped, located in Augusta, Michigan, is the world's largest riding school. This center has published an enthusiastically accepted, excellent training manual on therapeutic riding for the handicapped.

Disabled riders also can participate in riding clubs, especially in social and organizational capacities. They can easily assist at horse shows (by judging, for instance). Finally, there are carefully graded competitions for the disabled, devised in the Scandinavian countries and widely copied elsewhere.

Water sports have their own special attraction for many disabled people. Some water sports that are safely pursued by the handicapped include fly, float, and deep-sea fishing, canoeing, kayaking, rowing, sculling, sailing, waterskiing, motorboating, snorkeling, and scuba diving.

It is unfortunate that the potential benefit of water sports to be derived by the disabled is not more widely recognized. Fishing, which can be as simple or complicated as the angler chooses, can provide a thrilling awareness of the natural environment. It also can easily be enjoyed from a wheelchair or deck chair. A harness or fixed viselike pole-holder allows for one-handed fishing. Special lightweight rods, spinning reels, and other devices for the handicapped fisherman are available through catalogs and customer service personnel from several companies, including Orvis Co. (Manchester, Vt.) and L.L. Bean (Freeport, Me.). Sailing and canoeing are more risky than fishing, a characteristic that most youngsters and some older people find very stimulating.

It is the awareness of a new sense of freedom that is perhaps the greatest reward experienced by the disabled who participate in water sports. For those with restricted movement, involvement in watersports is another dimension of their lives in which the frustrations and difficulties of walking can be forgotten.

We now live in an era of supersophisticated technology. For the disabled, this certainly is beneficial. One of the most technical, competitive recreational activities available to the handicapped, particularly the quadriplegic, is target shooting. Two physicians from the Sheba Medical Center, Tel-Hashomer, Israel, devised a new flexible, spring-coil, multidirectional mounting device enabling competitive target shooting for individuals with severe bilateral upper- and lower-extremity physical handicaps, and even proposed rules based on the severity of paraplegia.

Of all disabled individuals, amputees are perhaps the people for whom the widest range of sports is possible. Indeed, a single, partial, upper-limb amputee is little disabled for running, race walking, speed skating, throwing the javelin, shot-putting, table tennis, and a number of other pursuits. Of the lower-limb amputees, below-knee amputees are significantly more independent than above-knee and bilateral amputees. (There is essentially no difference between above-knee and bilateral amputees.) Lower-limb amputees list fishing and swimming among the most popular recreational activities, whereas running and walking long distances head their list of the most arduous exercises. As might be anticipated, it is as true for the lower-limb amputee as it is for the able-bodied that as age increases, functional independence decreases.

Opportunities for Competition

For paraplegics, the wheelchair becomes their legs. Organized competitions in archery, basketball, badminton, bowling, croquet, darts, fencing, discus, golf, horseshoes, table tennis, pool, riflery, and road races (including marathons) have been arranged. Other leisure pursuits from square dancing to gardening can be enjoyed from the wheelchair seat. It is recommended that wheelchairs used for outdoor sports have removable arms, swinging or removable footrests, antitrip levers, outer hand rims, and, when desired, pneumatic tires.

It is suggested that disabled individuals who become deeply interested in competition contact the International Organization for the Disabled (Aylesbury, England), as various meets are held regularly on regional, national, and international levels. The U.S. National Wheelchair Games and International Paralympics are held annually and include events such as shot-putting, wheelchair track dashes and relays, weight lifting, archery, table tennis, swimming, and basketball. International Organization for the Disabled aims to unite national groups in international cooperation, to encourage further development of sports programs, and to provide a forum for the exchange of opinions, experiences, and resources related to sports for the disabled. It also prepares and disseminates international standards, so that individuals are divided into disability classifications to permit fair competition between participants with similar degrees of handicaps.

Some wheelchair athletes have made their competitive sport the focus of their life. Bob Hall of Belmont, Massachusetts, is a good example. A previous winner of the Boston Marathon and four other marathons in the wheelchair division, Hall began training in November for the April 1983 Boston Marathon. When the winter cold hit Boston, Hall moved to Florida for his twice-daily workouts of 8 to 12 mi. Once each week he "ran" 26 to 29 mi. at a pace of 6.33 to 7 min/mi. Midweek, he usually also wheeled one semilong run of 18 to 20 mi. Weekly, he covered an average of approximately 135 mi. with a maximum of 185 mi. Since Florida is primarily flat, Hall went to Bermuda to train for hill climbing and wind conditions. He also included in his exercise program short (30-minute), high-intensity, Nautilus weight training workouts two or three times weekly.

With such ability and commitment to training, one might think Bob Hall would be unbeatable. However, as skilled as he is, he did not win the 1983 Boston Marathon. Rather, 30-year-old Ken Archer, from Akron, Ohio, won the wheelchair event in 2 hours 38 minutes 59 seconds, 1 minute ahead of George Murray of Tampa, Florida. When the winter ice and cold came to Ohio, Archer took his training indoors, using a treadmill for his daily workouts. Faithful adherence to his conditioning routine resulted in his victory. Ironically, it was Bob Hall who sparked Archer's interest in wheelchair marathons. Archer says of wheelchair marathoning, "I do it because it gives me personal satisfaction."

How to Arrange One's Own Exercise Program

The basic requirements of an exercise program for the disabled are the same as those for the nondisabled. Each exercise program should have three parts: a warm-up period, an endurance phase, and a cooling-off period.

The warm-up period should be at least 5 minutes long and include rhythmic, slow, stretching movements of the trunk and limb muscles, preparing the body for sustained activity. To ignore the warm-up is to risk pulled muscles or more severe injuries.

The endurance phase should last at least 30 minutes. During this period, the cardiovascular system is stressed to increase aerobic capacity. To achieve maximal cardiovascular improvement, one should exercise vigorously enough during the endurance phase to be breathing deeply but not falling into greater oxygen debt (gasping for air). As an athlete's aerobic capacity increases, he or she may wish to increase the time and intensity of the endurance phase.

The cooling-off period too often is omitted in exercise. During the endurance phase, the body temperature is raised and the heart rate and blood pressure are increased considerably. Also in the endurance phase, lactic acid and other waste products build up in the muscles. The cooling-off phase allows the bodily functions gradually to return to normal. This helps to eliminate waste products from the muscles, minimizing the chance of stiffness and soreness the next day. The cooling-off period should last at least 5 minutes and can be longer if desired. It should include gross body movements that emphasize range of motion of the joints (calisthenics are ideal for this final step in the day's exercise program).

For the main endurance phase, I have prepared three lists of recreational pursuits that are easily adaptable to the upper-limb disabled (Table 3-1), lower-limb disabled (Table 3-2), and upper- and lower-limb disabled (Table 3-3). Those sports for which 30 minutes of continuous activity is

Table 3–1
Recreational Pursuits Especially Appropriate for the
Upper-Limb Disabled

Backpacking	Platform tennis
Badminton	Rodeo
Bicycling[a]	Roller skating[a]
Bowling	Running[a]
Cross-country running[a]	Snowshoeing
Darts	Soccer[a]
Fencing	Squash[a]
Horseback riding	Table tennis
Ice hockey[a]	Tennis
Ice skating[a]	Track
Jogging[a]	Trampoline[a]
Jumping[a]	Tumbling
Karate	Walking
Lawn bowling	

Source: Modified from Cantu, R.C. *Toward Fitness*. New York: Human Sciences Press, 1980, p. 120.
[a]Sports for which 30 minutes of continuous activity is sufficient.

sufficient are marked with a superscript letter *a*. Unmarked activities are those that are less strenuous, requiring an hour or more of participation per exercise period. It must be realized, though, that these tables are neither complete nor exclusive. For the highly motivated disabled individual with ingenuity, virtually any leisure or recreational activity can be mastered.

Table 3–2
Recreational Pursuits Especially Appropriate for the
Lower-Limb Disabled

Archery (W)	Lawn bowling (W)
Badminton (W)[a]	Motocross
Baseball (W)	Motorcycling
Basketball (W)[a]	Pool (W)
Boating	Rowing[a]
Body building (W)	Sailplanes
Bowling (W)	Show jumping
Canoeing[a]	Softball (W)
Folk dancing (W)	Sculling[a]
Football (touch or flag) (W)	Table tennis (W)
Gliding	Tobogganing
Golf	Volleyball (W)[a]
Handball (W)[a]	Weight lifting (W)
Kayaking[a]	

Source: Modified from Cantu, R.C. *Toward Fitness*. New York: Human Sciences Press, 1980, p. 121.
(W) denotes use of wheelchair.
[a]Sports for which 30 minutes of continuous activity is sufficient.

Table 3–3
Recreational Pursuits Enjoyed by Upper- and
Lower-Limb Disabled

Alpine skiing	Hunting
Body surfing[a]	Ice fishing
Bowling	Isometrics
Calisthenics	Rock climbing
Camping	Sailing
Cross-country skiing[a]	Scuba diving
Dancing	Skin diving
Darts	Skydiving
Diving (platform)	Snorkeling
Fishing	Sports car rallying
Gardening	Swimming[a]
Gymnastics	Target shooting
Hiking	Table tennis
Horseback riding	Waterskiing[a]

Source: Modified from Cantu, R.C. *Toward Fitness*. New York: Human Sciences
Press, 1980, p. 122.

[a]Sports for which 30 minutes of continuous activity is sufficient.

Appendixes to this chapter provide information about some of the
many athletic organizations for the disabled, as well as a selected
bibliography. Physically handicapped athletes are encouraged to arrange
their own exercise program and to use these resource lists fully.

Appendix 1: Athletic Organizations for the Disabled

Blind

1. American Blind Bowling Association
    150 North Bellaire Avenue
    Louisville, Kentucky 40206
    Phone: (502) 896-8039
    James Murrell, Secretary-Treasurer
    Founded: 1951. *Members:* 2600. *Regional groups:* 3. *Local groups:*
    130. Legally blind men and women, 18 years of age and older, com-
    peting in organized tenpin bowling. Promotes bowling as a recreational
    activity for adult blind people. Sponsors member leagues. Runs a yearly
    mail-o-graphic. Sponsors annual championship blind bowling tourna-
    ment; presents awards. *Publications: The Blind Bowler*, three issues
    yearly. *Convention/Meeting:* Annual tournament, May—1979,
    Cleveland, Ohio; 1980, Cincinnati, Ohio.

This list of organizations appeared previously in R.C. Cantu, *Toward Fitness*, New York:
Human Sciences Press, 1980, pp. 123–133. It is reprinted here, with minor editorial changes,
by permission.

2. Blind Outdoor Leisure Development
   533 East Main Street
   Aspen, Colorado 81611
   Phone: (303)925-8922
   Richard C. Fenton, Executive Director

   Founded: 1969. *Members:* 20. Operates on the "can-do" theory for blind people. Aids in the establishment of local clubs to enable the blind to experience the outdoors by skiing, skating, hiking, fishing, horseback riding, golfing, swimming, camping, and bicycling. Designs and conducts training courses for activity leaders. Has designed distinctive jackets and bibs to identify participants as blind. Provides insurance program for participants. Local clubs solicit reduced costs for, or free use of, sports equipment and facilities.

Deaf

1. American Athletic Association For The Deaf (AAAD)
   3916 Lantern Drive
   Silver Spring, Maryland 20902
   Phone: (301) 942-4042
   Richard Caswell, Secretary-Treasurer

   Founded: 1945. *Members:* 13,500. *Regional groups:* 7. *Local groups:* 155. Fosters athletic competition among the deaf and regulates uniform rules governing such competition. Provides adequate competition for those members who are primarily interested in interclub athletics. Provides a social outlet for deaf members and their friends. Sanctions and promotes state, regional, and national basketball tournaments, softball tournaments, and participation in activities of the Comite International des Sports Silencieux and in World Games for the Deaf. Maintains AAAD Hall of Fame and gives annual Athlete of the Year Award. *Publications:* Bulletin, quarterly. *Convention/Meeting:* Semiannual (April and September)—1979, Houston, Texas, and Cleveland, Ohio; 1980, San Diego, California, and Indianapolis, Indiana; 1981, Buffalo, New York, and Hartford, Connecticut; 1982, Miami, Florida, and Vancouver, British Columbia, Canada.

2. International Committee of the Silent Sports
   Gallaudet College
   Washington, D.C. 20002
   Phone: (202) 447-0841
   Jerald M. Jordan, Executive Secretary

Founded: 1924. *Members:* 43. Membership composed of athletic organizations for the deaf in each of 43 countries. Provides an international sports competition for the deaf, patterned after the International Olympic Games. Seeks to promote and develop physical education in general, and the practice of sports in particular, among the deaf. Encourages friendly relations between countries with programs in silent sports, and formation of silent sports programs in countries not yet participating. Holds Summer World Games and Winter Games alternately at 2-year intervals; all competitors must have severe hearing loss; awards gold, silver, and bronze medals to first, second, and third place winners of each event; medals recognizing valuable personal contribution to the Committee also are awarded. The Committee is recognized by the International Olympic Committee. *Publications:* Bulletin, quarterly; Handbook, irregular. *Convention/Meeting:* Biennial congress, held concurrently with Games.

3. United States Deaf Skiers Association
    159 Davis Avenue
    Hackensack, New Jersey 07601
    Dan Fields, President

Founded: 1968. *Members:* 310. Promotes skiing, both recreational and competitive, among the deaf and hearing-impaired in the United States. Provides deaf skiers benefits, activities, and opportunities which will further increase their enjoyment of the sport. Encourages ski racing among the deaf and sponsors national and regional races for deaf skiers. Assists in any way possible in the selection, organization, and training of the U.S. Deaf Ski Teams for international competition, such as in hockey, and the World Winter Games for the Deaf. Presents awards. *Committees:* Ice Figure Skating; Speed Skating. *Publications:* Newsletter, four yearly. *Affiliated with* U.S. Ski Association. *Convention/Meeting:* Biennial—February 1980, Steamboat Springs, Colorado; 1982, Big Sky, Montana.

Paralysis or Limbs Amputation

1. National Foundation For Happy Horsemanship For
    The Handicapped
    Box 462
    Malvern, Pennsylvania 19355
    Phone: (215) 644-7414
    Maudie Hunter-Warfel, National Adviser

Founded: 1967. Individuals who assist handicapped persons in their involvement with horses as a form of therapy and rehabilitation. Purpose is to encourage and unify the teaching of driving horses to the disabled through the training of personnel, and the arranging of exchanges among those who have experience in the field. Provides horses and donates facilities for their care. Provides films and conducts how-to clinics for volunteers. Maintains 200-volume library. *Councils:* National Advisory. *Publications:* Newsletter, annual. *Convention/ Meeting:* Biennial—September 1979, England.

2. National Handicapped Sports And Recreation Association
    4105 East Florida Avenue, Third Floor
    Denver, Colorado 80222
    Fred T. Nichol, President

    Founded: 1972. *Members:* 2207. *Local groups:* 13. Amputees and other handicapped persons who are interested in participating in all kinds of sports. Provides veterans and other inconvenienced (handicapped) persons an opportunity to experience sports and participatory recreation activities. Sponsors ski clinics and publishes an amputee ski technique manual. *Publications:* Bulletin, seminannual; also publishes *Amputee Ski Technique Manual* and *Blind Ski Teaching Manual. Formerly:* (1972) National Amputee Skiers Association; (1977) National Inconvenienced Sportsmen's Association. *Convention/Meeting:* Annual.

3. National Wheelchair Athletic Association (Handicapped) (NWAA)
    40–42 62nd Street
    Woodside, New York 11377
    Phone: (212) 424-2929
    Benjamin H. Lipton, Chairman

    Founded: 1958. *Members:* 1600. *Regional groups:* 13. Male and female athletes with significant permanent neuromusculoskeletal disability (spinal cord disorder, poliomyelitis, amputation) who compete in various amateur sports events in wheelchairs. The Association is administered by, and under the jurisdiction of the National Wheelchair Athletic Committee. Members compete in regional events and in the annual National Wheelchair Games, which include competitions in track and field (including pentathalon), swimming, archery, table tennis, slalom, and weightlifting. Qualifying rounds are held in each region to select competitors for the national competition. Selection is made at the completion of the nationals to represent the United States team in international competition. Travel expenses for the United States competitors are subsidized by the U.S. Wheelchair Sports Fund. *Publications:* Newsletter, quarterly.

4. National Wheelchair Basketball Association
    110 Seaton Building

University of Kentucky
Lexington, Kentucky 40506
Phone: (606) 257-1623
Stan Labanowich, Ph.D., Commissioner
Founded: 1958. *Members:* 130. *Conferences:* 24. Wheelchair basketball teams made up of individuals with severe permanent physical disabilities of the lower extremities. Seeks to provide opportunities on a national basis for the physically disabled to participate in the sport of wheelchair basketball, with its adjunct psychological, social, and emotional benefits, and to maintain a high level of competition through continuing refinement and standardization of playing rules and officiating. Sponsors competitions. Maintains hall of fame. Compiles statistics. Participates in charitable activities. Awards trophy annually to winner of National Wheelchair Basketball Tournament. *Publications: Weekly Standings and Statistics* (November-April); *Newsletter* biweekly (November–April); *Casebook*, annual; *Directory*, annual; *National Wheelchair Basketball Tournament Program*, annual; *Rules Book*, annual. *Convention/Meeting:* Annual sectional and regional tournaments leading up to the national tournament.

5. North American Riding For The Handicapped Association
    P.O. Box 100
    Ashburn, Virginia 22011
    Phone: (703) 777-3540
    Leonard Warner, Secretary-Treasurer

    Founded: 1968. *Members:* 200. Individuals and centers for the handicapped. Seeks to promote therapeutic riding for the handicapped, with safety and proper care, and to provide appropriate training and certification for instructors working with the handicapped. Makes periodic inspections of riding centers in operation. Provides consultants as lecturers and demonstrators. *Publications:* Newsletter, annual.

6. Special Olympics
    1701 K Street, N.W., Suite 203
    Washington, D.C. 20006
    Phone: (202) 331-1346
    Eunice Kennedy Shriver, President

    Founded: 1968. *Members:* 1,000,000. *Local groups:* 14,000. *Regional groups:* 8. *State groups:* 52. Created and sponsored by the Joseph P. Kennedy, Jr., Foundation to promote physical education and athletics for the retarded. Local, area, and chapter games are conducted in 50 states, District of Columbia, Puerto Rico, and 24 foreign countries. International Special Olympics are staged quadrennially (next: 1983). Participants range in age from 8 years to adult, and compete in track and field, swimming, gymnastics, bowling, ice skating, basketball,

and other sports. Information materials are available on organization
of programs and participation of athletes. Presents annual awards for
service to program through sports. Maintains speakers bureau. Compiles statistics. Sponsors research programs. *Councils:* National Advisory. *Publications:* Newsletter (restricted circulation), quarterly; List
of Chapter and National Directors, annual; also publishes brochure,
guide, instructional manual, and list of state programs. *Conven-
tion/Meeting:* Annual conference of chapter and national directors—August 9–12 1979, Brockport, New York.
7. American Coalition of Citizens with Disabilities
    1346 Connecticut Avenue, N.W.
    Washington, D.C. 20036
    Phone: (202) 785–4265

Appendix 2: Bibliography of Recreational Activities for the Handicapped

Archery

Heath, E.G.   *A History of Target Archery*, Devonshire, England: David
     and Charles Newton Abbott, 1973.

Camping

Summer camps for deaf children. *Alexander Graham Bell,* Association for
     the Deaf.   *Volta Rev.* 64:192–199, 1962.
Bauman, M.K., Strausse, S.   A comparison of blind children from day
     and residential schools in a camp setting. *Int. J. Educ. Blind* 11:74–77,
     1962.
Day Camping for the Cerebral Palsied. New York: United Cerebral Palsy
     Associations, Inc. Program Bulletin 11.
Frampten, M.E., Mitchell, P.C.   *Camping for Blind Youth.* New York:
     American Institute for the Education of the Blind, 1949.
Ginglend, D., Gould, K.   *Day Camping for the Mentally Retarded.* New
     York: National Association for Retarded Children, 1962.
Howett, H.H. (ed.)   *Camping for Crippled Children.* Chicago: National
     Society for Crippled Children and Adults, 1945.
Kapurch, J.A.   Camping though handicapped. *Am. J. Nurs.* 66:1794–
     1797, 1966.
Meyers, T.   *Camping for Emotionally Disturbed Boys.* Bloomington:
     Indiana University, Dept. of Recreation, School of Health, Physical
     Education, and Recreation, 1961.

Schoenbohm, W.F. *Planning and Operating Facilities for Crippled Children*. Springfield, Ill.: Charles C Thomas, 1962.

Switzer, R.M., Clark, M. Camping for severely disabled children. *Interclin. Information Bull*. 1964.

Gardening

Chaplin, M. *Gardening for the Physically Handicapped and Elderly*. Hippocrene Books, Batsford, 1978.

Wilshire, E.R. Equipment for the disabled. *Leisure and Gardening*, 2 Foredown Drive, Portsdale, Brighton BN4 2BB, England.

General

Adapted Sports, Games, Square Dances and Special Events. Hartford, Conn.: Connecticut Society for Crippled Children and Adults.

Adapted Sports in Veterans Administration. Special Services Information Bulletin 1B 6-252. Washington, D.C.: Recreation Service, U.S. Veterans Administration.

Barnett, M.W. Blind girl in the troop. *Girl Scout Leader*, April 1966, pp. 20-24.

Barnett, M.W. *Handicapped Girls and Girl Scouting: A Guide for Leaders*. New York: Girl Scouts of America, 1968.

Becker, E.F. *Female Sexuality Following Spinal Cord Injury*. Bloomington, Ill.: Accent Spinal Publishing.

Buell, C.E. Developments in physical education for blind children. *N. Outlook Blind* 58:202-206, 1964.

Buell, C.E. *Physical Education for Blind Children*. Springfield, Ill.: Charles C Thomas, 1966.

Davies, E.M. Let's get moving: Group activation of elderly people. *Age Concern*, 60 Pitcain Road, Mitcham, Surrey, England, 1975.

Dendy, E. Recreation for disabled people—what do we mean. *Physiotherapy* 64:290-291, 1978.

Emes, C. Physical work capacity of wheelchair athletes. *Res. Q. Am. Assoc. Health Phys. Educ.* 48:209-212, 1977.

Fait, H.F. *Adapted Physical Education*. Philadelphia: W.B. Saunders, 1960.

Glazier, R. (ed.). *The College Guide for Students with Disabilities*. Cambridge, Mass.: Abt Books, 1976.

Guttman, L. *Textbook of Sport for the Disabled*. Aylesbury, England: HM&M Publishers, 1976.

Holidays for the Physically Handicapped. Royal Association for Disability and Rehabilitation Annual, 1978 ed.

Howe, G.T.   Canoe course for the blind. *Recreation* 55:131–133, 1962.

Juul, K.D.   European approaches and innovations in serving the handicapped. *Except. Child* 44:322–330, 1978.

Kegel, B.; Carpenter, M.L., Burgess, E.M.   Functional capabilities of lower extremity amputees. *Arch. Physiol. Med. Rehab.* 59:109–120, 1978.

Kirchman, M.M.   Rifle holder. *Am. J. Occup. Ther.* 19:28, 1965.

Obe, N.C.   Outdoor activities. *Physiotherapy* 64:294–295, 1978.

Ohry, A., Talmor, E.   A new flexible spring-coil, multi-directional mounting device (with proposal of rules) for target shooting by the disabled. *Paraplegia Life* 16:5–7, 1978.

Paraplegia Life. Published by National Spinal Cord Injury Foundation, 369 Elliot St., Newton Upper Falls, Mass. 02164.

Rathbone, J.L., Lucus, C.   *Recreation in Total Rehabilitation*. Springfield, Ill.: Charles C Thomas, 1959.

Recreation for disabled people. *Physiotherapy* 64:299–301, 1978.

Sports and Spokes, 4330 East-West Highway, Suite 300, Washington, D.C. 20014.

Stewart, F.   *Recreation for the Retarded: A Handbook for Leaders*. London: National Society of Mentally Handicapped Children, 1975.

Swannell, A.J.   Medical considerations. *Physiotherapy* 64:292–293, 1978.

Taggie, J.M., Manley, M.S.   *A Handbook on Sexuality After Spinal Cord Injury*. Englewood, Colo.: Family Service Dept., Craig Hospital.

Travelability: A Guide for Physically Disabled Travelers in the United States. New York: Macmillan, 1978.

Wakim, K.G., Elkins, E., Worden, R, Polley, H.   The effects of therapeutic exercise on peripheral circulation of normal and paraplegic individuals. *Arch. Physiol. Med. Rehab.* 30:86–95, 1949.

Walker, G.M.   Riding for the disabled. *Physiotherapy* 64:297, 1978.

Weller, M.F.   Scouting for handicapped girls. *Girl Scout Leader*, May 1963.

Swimming

Mooney, H.V.   Fabricating of fin prostheses for bilateral amputee. *Orthop. Prostheses Appl. J.* September 1966, pp. 221–222.

Register of swimming clubs and organized swimming sessions for the handicapped people. National Association of Swimming Clubs for the Handicapped. 1977–1978.

Reid, M.J.   *Handling the Disabled Child in Water*. Association of Pediatric Chartered Physiotherapists (APCP) Publications, England: Crowley West Sussex, 1976.

Sterling, B.   *Aquatics for the Handicapped.* New York: Hoffman Harris, 1958.

Swimming for the Cerebral Palsied. New York: United Cerebral Palsy Associations, Inc. Program Bulletin 10.

Swimming for the Handicapped Instructors Manual. Washington, D.C.: American National Red Cross.

Other Water Sports

Guide to Fishing Facilities for Disabled Anglers. Peterborough, England: National Anglers Council, 1978.

Roberto, K.   Water sports. *Physiotherapy* 64:296, 1978.

State of the Art. *National Recreational Boating for the Physically Handicapped.* Long Island, N.Y.: Human Resource Center.

Water Sports for the Disabled. Woking, Surrey, England: The Sports Council Advisory Panel, Royal Yachting Association, 1977.

4

A Study of Physiologic Parameters Before and After a Season of Wheelchair Basketball Competition

Denis M. Desjardins, M.S.

With the growing popularity of wheelchair sports, the effects of competition on the physical fitness of athletes has become a pertinent topic for research. The lack of scientific data for use by those who work with wheelchair athletes has been noted by Corcoran et al. [1]. Some studies have reported physiologic profiles of disabled individuals [2–7], and other studies have compared these individuals with able-bodied athletes and sedentary individuals [8–10]. Different types of physical training programs for disabled people have been identified to promote positive changes in (1) relative maximal oxygen uptake ($\dot{V}o_2$ max), oxygen pulse (O_2 pulse), maximum ventilation ($\dot{V}c$ max), and percent of body fat [11]; (2) absolute $\dot{V}o_2$ max, dynamic strength, and muscular endurance [12]; (3) submaximal heart rate, and absolute and relative peak $\dot{V}o_2$ [13]; and (4) absolute $\dot{V}o_2$ max and maximal workload [14]. Only one study could be found which investigated the effects of a season of competition on wheelchair basketball players [15]. However, for this study, a Cameron Heartometer and a sphygmograph were used for data collection, which made comparisons with other studies difficult.

The purpose of the present study was to describe anthropometric and physiologic changes occurring in wheelchair basketball players over the course of a season of competition. A secondary purpose of the study was to compare these athletes' level of physical fitness with that of other wheelchair-confined sedentary individuals.

Subjects

The subjects included six members of the Rhode Island Rhode Runners wheelchair basketball team and one member of the Connecticut Spoke Benders wheelchair basketball team. They ranged in age from 21 to 33 years and had been involved in wheelchair basketball an average of 5 years. Of the subjects, four were ambulatory with the use of crutches or a cane and three were confined to wheelchairs. The wheelchair-confined individuals spent an average of 14 hr/day in their wheelchairs. The disability characteristics and competitive classifications of the subjects are presented in Table 4–1.

Table 4–1
Disability Characteristics of Subjects

Subject	Age	Disability	Years in Wheelchair	Years Playing Wheelchair Basketball
1	22	Spina bifida	Ambulatory	3
2	25	Hip aplasia	Ambulatory	8
3	24	Paraplegia	10	10
4	21	Paraplegia	4	3
5	27	Paraplegia	5	2
6	21	Cerebral palsy	Ambulatory	7
7	33	Below-knee amputee	Ambulatory	5

The subjects reported an average training time of 6 hr/wk, including games. During the season, three of the subjects were involved in wheelchair propelling workouts, one was involved in weight training, and the remaining three subjects were inactive except for basketball. Immediately prior to the beginning of the season, two subjects participated in wheelchair propelling for distance, one subject was involved in boxing, and another played golf. Three of the subjects were inactive prior to the season.

Methods

The investigation followed a test-treatment-retest design. Preseason testing was conducted the week before the beginning of regular season play. Postseason tests were administered approximately 4 months later, during the week immediately following the last day of competition. During the season, the subjects involved in the study participated in 13 league contests. Games were held on weekends and were played in two 20-minute periods. Practices were held twice weekly in the evening and lasted an average of 90 minutes. Practices consisted of intrasquad scrimmages in game situations.

Test Protocol

On entering the laboratory, the subjects were familiarized with the equipment and test protocol and were given the informed consent form to read and sign. Each subject was asked to remove any excess clothing, prosthesis, and braces, and then to switch from his wheelchair to one attached to a platform on a balance scale. Total body weight and sitting height then were recorded from the scale. Percent of body fat and body density were assessed using Lange skin-fold calipers (Lange Calipers Mfg., Cambridge, Md.) according to the method described by Pollock et al [16]. Three skin-fold measurements were recorded at each of two sites—the chest and axilla—and the mean of each set of measurements was recorded.

A resting electrocardiogram was taken with the subject in the seated position. From this, resting heart rate was determined and a screening was performed for abnormal cardiac activity. A blood sample of 40 μl then was obtained from the subject's right earlobe to determine the resting blood lactate concentration.

Data for spirometry were obtained using a Jaeger pneumotachygraph (Erich Jaeger, Rockford, Ill.). The four parameters evaluated were tidal volume (VT), vital capacity (VC), forced expiratory volume in 1 second (FEV$_{1.0}$), and a maximal voluntary ventilation (MVV). The grip strength of the dominant hand was assessed using a Takei handgrip dynamometer (Takei and Co., Tokyo, Japan).

The exercise tests were performed on a Monark bicycle ergometer (Monark-Crescent AB, Varberg, Sweden) adapted for arm cranking. The procedures followed in the submaximal and maximal tests were those described by Zwiren and Bar-Or [10]. The duration of the submaximal test was 6 minutes, with the initial workload set at 75 kelopond meters per minute (kpm/min) and increased by 75 kpm/min every 2 minutes. The cranking rate was 50 rpm and was maintained using a metronome. Heart rate readings were taken during the final 10 seconds of each minute.

The workload for the maximal test was developed through extrapolation of submaximal heart rates so that the duration would be approximately 6 minutes. The arm cranking rate for the maximal test was 50 rpm. The initial workload was increased by 150 kpm/min every 2 minutes until the subject was fatigued and could no longer keep the cranking pace or when abnormal symptoms were present [18]. Heart rate readings were taken during the final 10 seconds of each minute. Samples of expired air were collected minute by minute and analyzed using Jaeger Ergo-Pneumotest Oxygen and Carbon Dioxide Test gas analyzers.

On completion of the maximal test, recovery heart rate was monitored for 5 minutes and oxygen uptake for 2 minutes. After 5 minutes, another 40-μl blood sample was obtained for the determination of maximal blood lactate concentration. Blood samples were analyzed for lactic acid concentration by an enzymatic method (Boehringer-Mannheim Corporation, Brookfield, Conn.). Lactacid and alactacid capacities were calculated according to the formulas reported by Fox [17].

Data was analyzed using a t test for correlated samples. Further analyses were done on an individual basis in examining for patterns between variables.

Results

Anthropometric Changes

Table 4–2 lists the preseason and postseason values, their difference, and the percentages of change over the course of the season for the anthropometric variables of sitting height, body weight, percent of body fat, lean body weight, and body density. No significant changes were found in these variables.

Pulmonary Function Changes

In Table 4–3, the preseason and postseason values, their difference, and the percentage of change over the course of the season for the pulmonary function variables—V_T, VC, $FEV_{1.0}$, and MVV—are given. Of these variables, only the change in V_T was found to be significant ($p \leq 0.02$).

Physiologic Function Changes

Table 4–4 lists the preseason and postseason values and their difference as well as the percentage of change over the course of the season for the physio-

Table 4–2
Mean Anthropometric Changes

Variable	Preseason	Postseason	Difference	% Difference
Sitting height (cm)	85.63	85.36	−0.27	−0.32
Body weight (kg)	67.43	67.33	−0.10	−0.15
Body fat (%)	16.25	16.83	0.58	3.57
Lean body weight (kg)	55.95	55.38	−0.57	−1.01
Body density (g/cc)	1.062	1.060	−0.002	−0.19

Table 4–3
Mean Pulmonary Function Changes

Variable	Preseason	Postseason	Difference	% Difference
Tidal volume (L)	0.88	0.69	−0.19	−21.14[a]
Vital capacity (L)	4.03	4.15	0.12	2.98
Forced expiratory volume in 1 sec (L)	3.29	3.23	−0.06	−1.82
Maximal voluntary ventilation (L/min)[b]	167.97	169.55	1.58	0.94

[a] $p < 0.02$.
[b] $n = 4$.

Table 4-4
Mean Physiologic Function Changes

Variable	Preseason	Postseason	Difference	% Difference
Grip strength (kg)	53.71	57.28	3.57	6.65
Maximal heart rate (beats/min)	186.14	185.28	−0.86	−0.46
Maximal oxygen uptake				
Absolute (L/min)	2.05	1.94	−0.11[a]	−5.37
Relative (ml/kg · min)	31.26	29.37	−1.89[b]	−6.05
Oxygen pulse (ml/beat)	11.06	10.48	−0.58	−5.24
Maximal ventilation (L/min)	86.27	83.11	−3.16	−3.66

[a]$p \leq 0.05$.
[b]$p \leq 0.01$.

logic function variables of grip strength, maximal heart rate, absolute and relative $\dot{V}o_2$ max, O_2 pulse, and $\dot{V}e$ max. Among these variables, significant decreases were found in absolute $\dot{V}o_2$ max ($p \leq 0.05$) and relative $\dot{V}o_2$ max ($p \leq 0.01$).

Metabolic Function Changes

The preseason and postseason values, their difference, and the percentage of change over the course of the season for the metabolic function variables are given in Table 4-5. These variables include caloric production of the aerobic system, lactacid capacity, alactacid capacity, and maximum blood lactate concentration. Of these, only the decrease in the caloric production of the aerobic system was found to be significant ($p \leq 0.01$). This was expected since this variable is derived directly from the relative $\dot{V}o_2$ max.

Discussion

This study failed to find any favorable physical changes in the subjects over the course of a season of wheelchair basketball competition. An examination

Table 4-5
Mean Metabolic Function Changes

Variable	Preseason	Postseason	Difference	% Difference
Maximal oxygen intake (calories/kg · min)	156.29	146.87	−9.42[a]	−6.05
Lactacid capacity (calories/kg)	140.77	101.23	−39.54	−28.09
Alactacid capacity (calories/kg)	36.78	30.31	−6.47	−17.59
Maximal blood lactate concentration (mM/L)[b]	9.92	7.18	−2.74	−27.62

[a]$p \leq 0.01$.
[b]$n = 5$.

tion of the anthropometric variables revealed no patterns of change among the subjects. The insignificant changes that were found in these variables could be due to the diet or degree of activity engaged in by the individual, neither of which were controlled during the study. It is believed that training during the season, although not quantified, was not intense enough to elicit significant positive changes.

Bar-Or et al. [13] also reported no change following a 12-month mild conditioning program. This program was conducted twice per week in sessions lasting 2 hours. The intensity of the program was not quantified. Pollock et al. [11], however, reported significant reductions in percent of body fat of disabled individuals after a 20-week training program. In this program, training sessions were conducted three times per week and lasted 30 minutes. Training heart rates averaged between 155 and 165 beats per minute.

The significant decrease found in V_T may be attributable to the subjects' familiarity with the test procedure during the postseason evaluation. No other pulmonary function variable showed a significant change.

Post season evaluations revealed significant decreases in both absolute and relative $\dot{V}o_2$ max. Since both duration (4 months) and frequency (three times per week, including games) of the training sessions were sufficient to produce positive changes, it is believed the intensity was not. Again, the intensity of each session was not quantified.

Data representing the physiologic function of each subject was examined with respect to the individual's activity prior to the season. It was found that those subjects who were inactive (Patients 3, 5, and 6) exhibited the lowest preseason values for absolute and relative $\dot{V}o_2$ max, O_2 pulse, and MVV, as shown in Table 4-6. On completion of the season, these subjects had not improved and still were ranked the lowest in the group. This data further supports the assumption that training during the season of competition was not intense enough to elicit significant positive changes in the variables studied.

Table 4-6
Maximal Oxygen Uptake ($\dot{V}o_2$ max) for Each Subject

Subject	Absolute $\dot{V}o_2$ (L/min)		Relative $\dot{V}o_2$ max (ml/kg · min)	
	Preseason	Postseason	Preseason	Postseason
1	2.32	2.26	38.3	37.4
2	2.96	2.83	29.3	28.3
3	1.85	1.83	26.7	27.0
4	2.26	2.29	48.3	45.7
5	1.61	1.39	24.0	21.2
6	1.21	1.07	23.5	20.5
7	2.16	1.93	28.7	25.5

Lactacid capacity and alactacid capacity were derived from formulas reported by Fox [17]. Since there is still some question as to the validity and reliability of these formulas for use in studies in which arm cranking is the exercise modality, this data is presented with some reservation. Fox reported mean values obtained for able-bodied college-aged men to be 200 calories/kg for lactacid capacity and 100 calories/kg for alactacid capacity. In comparison, values obtained in the present study were found to be low.

In summary, it was found that the physical fitness levels of the subjects involved in this study were not significantly improved. This was reflected by decreases in each of the physiologic and metabolic parameters evaluated. Smith [15] reported a similar decrease in conditioning levels toward the end of a season of competition and attributed it to competitive fatigue and tension. The results obtained in the present study could be due to a gradual detraining over the course of the season or to factors such as those reported by Smith. However, such factors could not be quantified owing to the limited test data available.

The low number of subjects and the lack of uniformity in the disability characteristics of the subjects in this study places a limitation on the results obtained. Another limitation is that only preseason and postseason test data were recorded. Therefore, a longitudal study with a larger and more uniform subject pool should be undertaken. Such a longitudinal study should include testing at predetermined intervals over the course of 1 year, with a complete inventory of the subjects' activity patterns during that time. It could yield valuable information concerning fitness levels prior to preseason training, at some point following the completion of the season, and during various seasons of the year. This information could, in turn, be used by those who coach and promote wheelchair basketball competition.

References

1. Corcoran, P.J., Goldman, R.F., Hoerner, E.F., et al. Sports medicine and the physiology of wheelchair marathon racing. *Orthop. Clin. North Am.* 11:697–716, 1980.
2. Cameron, B.J., Ward, C.R., Wicks, J.R. Relationship of type of training to maximum oxygen uptake and upper limb strength in male paraplegic athletes (abstract). *Med. Sci. Sports Exerc.* 9:58, 1977.
3. Gandee, R., Winningham, M., Deitchman, R., Narraway, R. The aerobic capacity of an elite wheelchair marathon racer (abstract). *Med. Sci. Sports Exerc.* 12:142, 1980.
4. Gass, C.C., Camp, C.M. Physiological characteristics of trained Australian paraplegic and tetraplegic subjects. *Med. Sci. Sports Exerc.* 11:256–259, 1979.

5. Hjeltnes, N.   Oxygen uptake and cardiac output in graded arm exercise in paraplegics with low level spinal cord lesions. *Scand. J. Rehabil. Med.* 9:107–113, 1977.

6. Taylor, A.W., Royer, D., Steadward, R., et al.   Skeletal muscle analysis of wheelchair athletes (abstract). *Med. Sci. Sports Exerc.* 11:114, 1979.

7. Wicks, J.R., Head, E., Oldridge, N.B., et al.   Maximum oxygen uptake of wheelchair athletes competing at the 1976 Olympiad for the Physically Disabled (abstract). *Med. Sci. Sports Exerc.* 9:58, 1977.

8. Emes, C.   Physical work capacity of wheelchair athletes. *Res. Q. Exerc. Sport* 48:209–212, 1977.

9. Heigenhauser, G.F., Ruff, G.L., Miller, B., Faulkner, J.A.   Cardiovascular response of paraplegics during graded arm ergometry (abstract). *Med. Sci. Sports Exerc.* 8:68, 1976.

10. Zwiren, L.D., Bar-Or, O.   Responses to exercise of paraplegics who differ in conditioning level. *Med. Sci. Sports Exerc.* 7:94–98, 1975.

11. Pollock, M.L., Miller, H.S., Linnerud, A.C. et al.   Arm pedaling as an endurance training regimen for the disabled. *Arch. Phys. Med. Rehabil.* 55:418–424, 1974.

12. Nilsson, S., Staff, P.H., Pruett, E.D.R.   Physical work capacity and the effects of training on subjects with long standing paraplegia. *Scand. J. Rehabil. Med.* 7:51–56, 1975.

13. Bar-Or, O., Inbar, O., Spira, R.   Physiological effects of a sports rehabilitation program on cerebral palsied and post-poliomyelitic adolescents. *Med. Sci. Sports Exerc.* 8:157–161, 1976.

14. Dreisinger, T.E., Londeree, B.R., Craig, H.W., et al.   Wheelchair ergometric training in the handicapped (abstract). *Med. Sci. Sports Exerc.* 11:112, 1979.

15. Smith, R.W.   The Progressive Preseason, Competitive, and Postseason Changes in Selected Physical Fitness Characteristics of Eleven Wheelchair Basketball Players. Master's thesis, University of Illinois, 1967.

16. Pollock, M.L., Wilmore, J.H., Fox, S.M.   *Health and Fitness Through Physical Activity.* New York: John Wiley and Sons, 1978.

17. Fox, E.L.   Differences in metabolic alterations with sprint versus endurance interval training programs. In Howald, H., Poortmans, J.R., (eds.), *Metabolic Adaptations to Prolonged Physical Exercise.* Basel: Birkhauser Verlag, 1975, pp. 119–126.

18. American College of Sports Medicine.   *Guidelines for Grades Exercise Testing and Exercise Prescription.* Philadelphia: Lea & Febiger, 1975.

5

Pulmonary and Cardiac Adjustments of Orthopedic Patients To A Mask-Flippers-Snorkel Aquatic Therapeutic Exercise Program

Thomas G. Manfredi, Ph.D.
Loretta DiPietro, M.S.
Michael Gavin, R.P.T., P.C.

People suffering from a variety of orthopedic disorders, including cerebral palsy, multiple sclerosis, arthritis, and postoperative conditions, find that water is a better therapeutic medium since they can perform movements in the water that cannot possibly be done on the treatment table. These people often do not exercise enough aerobically to obtain any cardiovascular benefits which offer protection against coronary heart disease.

The bouyancy effect of water causes the body to weigh approximately one-tenth its normal weight on land. The water medium offers unlimited range of motion and a low resistance to movement, and eliminates the gravitational effects of land exercises which often produce overwhelming forces on the spine, knees, and ankles. Warm water reduces pain in arthritic patients during exercise and produces a sedative effect, offering a valuable means of treating certain emotional or mental disorders. Exercise prescription for swimmers often is accomplished from graded exercise tests performed on a treadmill or bicycle ergometer. Prescribed target heart rates for swimming usually are 5 to 10 beats per minute lower than heart rates prescribed for running or bicycling.

The purpose of this study was to evaluate the effects of a 10-week mask, flippers, and snorkel (MFS) therapeutic swimming program on selected cardiac, pulmonary, and orthopedic measurements in orthopedic patients.

The Mask, Flippers, and Snorkel Therapeutic Program

The MFS program was originated in Milford, Connecticut, by Michael Gavin, a registered physical therapist.* The original intent of the program

The authors wish to acknowledge Mr. Stanley Gloss, Director of the Department of Respiratory Therapy, Quinnipiac College, Hamden, Connecticut, for his assistance in the pulmonary assessment of patients.
*Michael Gavin, R.P.T., P.C., 281 Seaside Avenue, Milford, Connecticut 06460.

was to provide an exercise modality for people with low back problems. The use of a mask, snorkel, and flippers has many advantages. The snorkel provides easy and steady breathing. It also minimizes or eliminates the Valsalva maneuver and diving reflex which sometimes occur from holding one's breath. The mask facilitates visibility to check on proper swimming technique under water. The mask and snorkel also serve to keep the neck in a relaxed position. The flippers allow the patient to move farther and faster in the water, thus facilitating movement while offering aerobic and musculoskeletal training effects not accomplished through faulty swimming technique. Finally, the use of this equipment enables the swimmer to modify any basic swimming stroke to best treat his or her individual weakness.

Prior to entering the swimming program, each patient is taught by specially trained instructors the correct techniques for using the mask, flippers, and snorkel approach to swimming. The swimming session is preceded by a warm-up period using exercises that facilitate maintenance of the pelvic tilt.

The patients are instructed to swim in a prone C position. This position rotates the upper part of the pelvis backward and minimizes strain which often is produced by increased lumbar lordosis. While in the C position, the head is relaxed with no neck extension. The subject is instructed to look at the bottom of the pool while moving his or her feet in a bicycle kick with hip flexion not exceeding a 90-degree angle. The advanced subjects use a combination flutter and bicycle kick below the surface of the water. Sculling is done by moving the forearms in a circular motion up toward the head.

Methods

The exercise program was conducted over a 10-week period using 10 participants from Gavin's MFS therapeutic classes. Static pulmonary measurements using a Collins 13-L spirometer (Warren E. Collins, Inc., Braintree, Mass.) were taken at the pool site during the first, fifth, and tenth week of the program. Six skin-fold sites also were measured during each testing session. The skin-fold sites used were the triceps, subscapular, pectoralis, umbilicus, iliac, and anterior thigh.

During each testing session, each participant was given a 12-minute swim-for-distance test. The distance in pool lengths covered during the swim was calculated. Also, each participant's pulse rate was monitored for 1 minute immediately following the swim.

All swimming classes were held in a pool 25 yd long, with the two end lanes approximately 4 ft deep along their entire length. The water temperature was maintained at approximately 80°F.

Results

Eight men and two women, aged 20 to 68 years, underwent a 10-week MFS program. The subjects are described in Table 5-1. Orthopedic dysfunctions included low back disorders in two subjects and one case each of a hip replacement, multiple sclerosis, paraplegia, and post-knee surgery. Four subjects had no dysfunctions.

Table 5-2 shows individual changes in body fat using a formula established by Jackson and Pollock [1]. Mean body weight dropped only 0.8 kg during the first 5 weeks and 1.2 kg between weeks 1 and 10. The values for percent of body fat changed very little during the 10-week swimming program. However, most of the loss in body weight was attributable to fat loss, with lean body weight remaining almost unchanged.

Table 5-3 summarizes the changes in selected pulmonary function tests throughout the 10-week study. A mean peak flow of 7.1 L/sec found prior to the swimming program was 29 percent below expected normal values. By week 5, the mean peak flow was 8.2 L/sec or 17 percent below normal values. No appreciable change was found in peak flow from weeks 5 to 10. Forced vital capacity (FVC) dropped during the first 5 weeks from 4.18 to 3.77 L and rose to 4.04 L at the end of 10 weeks. Percent of FVC for 0.5 seconds and 1.0 seconds increased appreciably during the first 5 weeks of the program and showed no real changes from weeks 5 to 10. Forced expiratory volume in 0.5 seconds ($FEV_{0.5}$) rose from 45.3 to 54.6 percent during the first 5 weeks and forced expiratory volume in 1 second ($FEV_{1.0}$) rose from 66.8 to 75 percent during this time, bringing both values within normal expected ranges.

Table 5-4 shows the results of a 12-minute swim-for-distance test and the mean recovery heart rates monitored for 1 minute immediately following the swim. The distances covered during the swim test were 393 yd, 545 yd, and 578 yd for weeks 1, 5, and 10 respectively, representing a 32 percent increase in yardage from week 1 to week 10. Mean recovery heart rates were 120 beats per minute during week 1 and 114 beats per minute during weeks 5 and 10. These data imply that the MFS program allows patients with coronary heart disease and orthopedic problems to exercise in a manner that is nearly impossible for them using other modalities, including conventional swimming, and brings about considerable physiologic changes within safe target heart rates.

Discussion

Although swimming appears to provide distinct advantages as a rehabilitative modality for cardiac and orthopedic disorders, there are still many

Table 5-1
Description of Subjects in Mask-Flippers-Snorkel Therapeutic Swimming Program

Subject	Sex	Age (yr)[a]	Dysfunction	Comments
1	M	35	Low back disorder	Smoker: one pack per day for 15 yr. Exercised 1–2 days/wk; poor tolerance of water due to low percent of body fat
2	M	20	Low back disorder	Exercised 1–2 days/wk. Stopped for 5 wk owing to poor tolerance of cold water. In the program 20 wk
3	M	60	Hip replacement	Exercised 3 times weekly for 27 wk. Swam up to 44 laps in 45 min. Highly motivated
4	M	38	Paraplegia	Exercised 1–2 days/wk for 2 yr
5	M	67	None	Exercised 3–4 times weekly for 11 wk. Swam 94 laps in 1 hr 5 min. Highly motivated
6	M	68	None	Exercised 3–4 times weekly for 11 wk. Swam 60 laps in 50 min. Highly motivated. Smoked, but stopped 15 yr before entering program
7	F	25	None	A swimmer. Ran 1–2 times weekly, 1–3 mi., 9 min/mi. In program for 11 wk; dieting
8	F	40	None	Exercised 4–5 times weekly. Stopped for 5 weeks. Highly motivated; dieting
9	M	56	Multiple sclerosis	Exercised once weekly for more than 1 yr
10	M	26	Knee disorder that required surgery	Exercised 3 times weekly for 10 wk

[a]Mean ± SD (43.5 ± 17.9).

Table 5-2
Individual and Mean Changes in Skin-fold Measurements, Percent of Body Fat, and Body Weight from Week 1 to Week 10

Subject	Week 1			Week 5			Week 10		
	Total of Skin-fold Measurements[a]	% Body Fat	Body Weight (kg)	Total of Skin-fold Measurements[a]	% Body Fat	Body Weight (kg)	Total of Skin-fold Measurements[a]	% Body Fat	Body Weight (kg)
1	38	6.0	64.9	33	6.0	64.4	35	6.0	63.7
2	36	4.0	61.2	36	4.0	60.8	36	4.0	59.5
3	180	32.0	98.9	186	32.7	98.0	153	28.6	98.0
4[b]									
5	111	22.7	77.1	101	20.6	77.6	101	20.6	76.2
6	116	23.8	70.3	110	22.7	69.9	119	23.8	69.9
7	112	18.1	59.9	108	18.1	58.1	89	14.8	57.7
8	154	26.0	78.0	133	23.2	74.0	148	25.1	74.0
9	95	20.6	82.6	91	19.4	83.5	88	19.4	83.5
10	90	14.8	70.3	87	14.8	69.9	80	13.6	69.9
Mean	114.7	18.7	73.7	98.3	17.9	72.9	94.3	17.3	72.5
±SD	52.7	8.6	11.5	44.0	8.3	11.6	40.0	8.0	11.9

[a]Skin-fold measurements were taken at the following six sites: triceps, subscapular, pectoralis, umbilicus, iliac, and anterior thigh.
[b]Unable to assess six skin-fold sites on this subject.

Table 5-3
Mean Changes in Pulmonary Measurements in Total Population from Week 1 to Week 10

Function	Weeks 1 through 5 (n = 10)				Weeks 1 through 10 (n = 9)		
	Week 1	Week 5	Difference from Week 1 to Week 5	% Difference from Week 1 to Week 5	Week 10	Difference from Week 1 to Week 10	% Difference from Week 1 to Week 10
Peak flow	7.1 L/sec ± 2.88	8.2 L/sec ± 3.38	+1.1 L/sec	13.5	8.3 L/sec ± 3.52	+1.2 L/sec	15.2
FVC	4.18 L ± 0.89	3.77 L ± 1.23	−0.41 L	−10	4.04 L ± 1.15	−0.14 L	−3.3
$FEV_{0.5}$ %	45.3% ± 18.3	54.6% ± 19.3	+9.4%	17	54.2% ± 23.1	+8.9%	16.5
$FEV_{1.0}$ (%)	66.8% ± 18.2	75% ± 18.7	+8.2%	11	75.6% ± 23.1	+8.9%	11.7
$FEV_{3.0}$ (%)	91.8% ± 10.9	96.6% ± 7.17	+4.9%	5	98.7% ± 4.05	+7.0%	7
$FEV_{0.5}$ (L)	1.82 L ± 0.819	2 L ± 0.82	+0.18 L	9	2.25 L ± 1.11	+0.44 L	19.2
$FEV_{1.0}$ (L)	2.8 L ± .887	2.82 ± 0.971	+0.02 L	0.8	2.82 L ± 1.01	+0.02 L	0.8
$FEV_{3.0}$ (L)	3.86 L ± 1.11	3.67 L ± 1.32	−0.19 L	−5	3.93 L ± 1.22	+0.07 L	1.8

FVC = forced vital capacity; FEV_x = forced expiratory volume in x seconds.

Table 5-4
Mean Changes in Cardiac Measurements (Twelve-Minute Swim Test) in Total Population[a]

Variable	Week 1	Week 5	Difference from Week 1 to Week 5	% Difference from Week 1 to Week 5	Week 10	Difference from Week 1 to Week 10	% Difference from Week 1 to Week 10
No. of laps swum	15.7 ± 10.9	21.8 ± 11.9	+6.2	28	23.1 ± 13.5	+7.4	32
Recovery heart rate (beats/min)	120 ± 20.4	114 ± 17.7	−6	−5	114 ± 14.95	−6	−5

[a] $n = 9$.

questions regarding the safety of swimming for cardiac patients. Cold-water immersion studies showed elevated resting heart rates and systolic blood pressure on entry [2], followed by decreases in heart rates and cardiac outputs along with inadequate ventricular filling [3]. Pool temperatures should be higher than 25°C or 77°F, with an optimal temperature ranging between 82° and 86°F.

Prone swimming, compared to equivalent land exercises, has been shown to increase minute ventilation, lower heart rate [4], raise stroke volumes, and lower ventilatory equivalents [5, 6]. Magder et al. [7] found occasional ectopic beats in a few of their nine cardiac patients on entering the water. Player and Blazek [8] found a lesser incidence of ST-segment depression in their cardiac patients who swam, compared to running, suggesting that swimming offers some kind of protection from ST-segment depression. They further concluded that the bradycardia dive reflex on submersion for 15 to 30 seconds occurs in a normal manner in cardiac patients, even with those on propranolol hydrochloride. The study by Heigenhauser et al. [9] concluded that swimming exercises can be safely prescribed from a graded exercise test performed on a bicycle ergometer. Wilson [10] suggests that target heart rates prescribed for swimming be approximately 5 beats per minute lower than targets prescribed for other forms of exercise, whereas McArdle et al. [11] suggest swimming intensities be prescribed at target values 13 beats per minute lower than running.

In conclusion, the mask, flippers, and especially the snorkel offer artificial aids for the exercise program participant which may effectively deal with the usual cardiac concerns specific to the water medium. Further investigation into the safety and efficacy of this program is urged.

References

1. Jackson, A.S., Pollock, M.L.   Generalized equation for predicting body density of man. *Br. J. Nutr.* 40:497–501, 1978.

2. Goode, R.C., Duffin, J., Miller, R., et al.   Sudden cold water immersion. *Respir. Physiol.* 23:301–310, 1975.

3. Nielsen, B.   Physiology of thermoregulation during swimming. In Eriksson, B., and Furberg, B. (Eds.), *Swimming Medicine,* vol. 4. Baltimore: University Park Press, 1978, pp. 297–304.

4. Kasch, F.W.   Maximal oxygen uptake in older male swimmers during free swimming and stationary cycling. In Eriksson B., and Furberg, B. (Eds.), *Swimming Medicine,* vol. 4. Baltimore: University Park Press, 1978.

5. Holmer, I., Stein, E.M., Saltin, B., et al.   Hemodynamic and respiratory responses compared in swimming and running. *J. Appl. Physiol.* 37:49–54, 1974.

6. McArdle, W.D., Glaser, R.M., Magel, S.R. Metabolic and cardiorespiratory responses during free swimming and treadmill walking. *J. Appl. Physiol.* 30:733, 1971.

7. Magder, S., Linnarsson, D., Gullstrand, L.   The effect of swimming on patients with ischemic heart disease. *Circulation* 63:5, 1981.

8. Player, J.S., Blazek, V.W.   A telemetry study of 9 cardiac patients while swimming and running. University of Illinois, Abraham Lincoln School of Medicine. Typescript.

9. Heigenhauser, G.F., Boulet, D., Miller, B., Faulkner, J.A.   Cardiac outputs of post-myocardial infarction patients during swimming and cycling. *Med. Sci. Sports* 9:143–147, 1977.

10. Wilson, P.K.   Water exercises for prevention, intervention, and rehabilitation from coronary artery disease. In Stadalis, R.E. (Ed.), *Research and Practices in Physical Education: Selected Papers from the 1976 Research Symposia of the American Alliance for Health, Physical Education, and Recreation National Convention.* Champaign, Ill.: Human Kinetics Publishers, 1976, pp. 147–155.

11. McArdle, W.D., Katch, F.I., Katch, V.L.   Training for anaerobic and aerobic power. In *Exercise Physiology: Energy, Nutrition, and Human Performance.* Philadelphia: Lea and Febiger, 1981, p. 276.

6

Handicapped Skiing: An Overview

David P. McCormick, M.D.

In recent years, recreational activities have become more available for disabled persons. Handicapped athletes now participate in a wide variety of activities, such as basketball, tennis, track, marathon running, and archery [1]. The disabled athlete experiences the same advantages through sports participation as does a nondisabled athlete. There is the joy of movement, the feeling of well-being that results from physical fitness, the exhilaration of competition, and the companionship and travel opportunities that derive from membership in an athletic team or club.

Primary care physicians, orthopedists, physical therapists, and others interested in sports medicine should be aware of handicapped skiing, a sport which has been popularized in recent years. Programs for the disabled at areas such as Winter Park in Colorado and Mt. Sunapee in New Hampshire have made skiing available to many disabled individuals. Advances in teaching techniques and adaptive equipment enable these individuals to ski successfully even though they may have significant physical limitations. A person with amputation of one or both lower extremities, with paresis of extremities, or with partial or complete blindness can ski safely when provided with the appropriate equipment and instruction. The disabled skier frequently progresses at a much slower rate in acquiring skills, but eventual mastery of the sport is accompanied by an understandable sense of accomplishment.

Physical Assessment

Handicapped skiing programs such as that organized by the New England Handicapped Sportsman's Association at Mt. Sunapee usually precede skiing lessons with a physical assessment of the prospective skier. The nature of the handicap is determined so that specialized equipment can be selected.

Lower-Extremity Amputation or Weakness

Lower-extremity amputees will need differing equipment depending on the level of amputation. Loss of the foot at the ankle usually will permit skiing on two skis with two poles in the usual fashion. The lower-leg prosthesis will almost always fit a normal ski boot. A strap from the top of the prosthesis to the skier's belt normally is worn to stabilize the prosthesis during turns or if a fall should occur. Without such a strap, the ski, boot, and prosthesis could fall off the leg when the skier is riding the lift.

Amputations above the ankle do not usually permit the skier to wear a weight-bearing prosthesis since there is insufficient control of the ski on the weak side. If the skier wears such a prosthesis, with or without a ski attached, a fall can result in significant stump injury, sometimes even severe enough to fracture the femur. For convenience, the above-knee amputee often will wear a lightweight socket-type prosthesis which accepts a removable pylon. The peg can be attached to the prosthesis for easy mobility between the ski lodge and lift areas at the bottom of the ski hill.

The above-knee amputee usually learns to ski well on one ski when provided with a set of outrigger ski poles. This combination is called *tri-track* or *three-track skiing*. The outrigger is a modified Canadian crutch with a ski tip attached. Various spring-assisted devices are available which permit the ski tip to snap up when the skier is walking. This feature is especially useful when the skier is negotiating uphill grades at the top and bottom of ski lifts.

As the tri-track skier's skill advances, less weight is applied to the outriggers and they are used more for balance and as a check while negotiating turns or moguls. Expert tri-trackers sometimes do away with the heavier outriggers and ski with standard ski poles. This technique requires superior balance, strength, and coordination. Easier terrain often is a necessity in this instance.

Although some disabled individuals may be able to walk on both legs, one leg may be too weak to control the added weight of a ski. Such people usually prefer the tri-track method with outrigger ski poles. The weak foot can be tethered to the opposite boot with a short length of shock cord, or the foot can be rested on a metal shelf projecting from the medial side of the opposite boot.

To obtain adequate control, people with bilateral lower-extremity weakness or amputation usually require two skis. Sometimes a so-called ski bra is needed. This device atttaches to the ski tips and allows the tips to be hooked together. The skis can thereby be stabilized in a wedge or snowplow position which aids control and maneuverability.

Individuals with bilateral above-knee or below-knee amputations or people with one above-knee and one below-knee amputation can ski in the upright position wearing prostheses if they also are provided with outriggers. This is called *four-track skiing*. Wedging of boots and special bent-knee prostheses sometimes are necessary to position the legs for adequate control. The skier turns primarily by shifting his or her upper body weight from side to side and by throwing a torque or rotational component into the upper body as the weight shifts.

Ski specifications often are important. The maneuverability of a ski depends on a number of factors, including ski length, weight, camber, stiffness, and width. A reverse camber rocker-bottom ski, which provides for easy initiation of turns, has been designed for use by handicapped skiers. Wider skis tend to be more stable and are more appropriate for beginners. More advanced skiers may prefer a longer, heavier, stiffer ski, which is more stable at high speeds, or a ski with a narrow waist, which provides more quickness from edge to edge.

Another method of skiing, *sit-skiing*, has become available for use in controlled situations with experienced instructors. The sit-ski is a sled designed for skiers whose lower-extremity strength and coordination are not capable of supporting upright skiing. The sit-ski has a leg cover for warmth and protection, a roll bar, runners which can be sharpened or waxed, and an evacuation device beneath the seat with rope and pully that enables a skier to lower himself or herself safely down from a ski lift in case of power failure. For additional safety, it always is necessary to tether the sit-skier to an expert instructor who followers behind. In case of emergency, the sit-skier can be brought to a stop by the safety tether. The ski itself is controlled not by the tether but by the skier. The ski is steered by a shifting of upper body weight and by poling against the snow with a single kayak-type ski pole or with separate very short ski poles held in each hand. The sit-ski has just been introduced for use in the eastern United States, and its eventual utility and popularity remain to be seen. It should be used only in approved areas under the guidance of expert assistants.

Visual Impairment

The visually impaired student may be totally or only partially blind. He or she may see well enough to follow close behind a guide who leads the way down the hill. Such skiers can successfully negotiate slalom courses. Brightly colored "blind skier" bibs always are worn by the guide and the student as a warning to other skiers. Totally blind skiers usually are followed down the hill by their guide who visually searches a pie-shaped area downhill while at the same time calling out instructions to the student. Blind skiers prefer familiar trails, and they like to work with the same guide from week to week.

Blind beginning skiers require a wide variety of instructional methods and enthusiastic instructors who are willing to improvise when necessary. Lessons begin with a thorough exploration by touch and feel of the skier's equipment—boots, poles, bindings, and skis. The student may need to hold the instructor's body while the positions and steering movements are demonstrated. Blind skiers, like other disabled skiers, must first learn to fall safely, since sometimes this is the only way to regain control in hazardous situations.

The Handicapped Skiers' Club

The largest and most active ski organization for disabled skiers in the Eastern United States is the New England Handicapped Sportsman's Association. Enthusiastic membership derives from the fact that most members are disabled. However, a large number of able-bodied individuals also participate. This promotes a healthy communication between disabled and able-bodied participants. By working closely, the members can develop a realistic appreciation for the special needs of others in the group. New members are treated with a caring approach, but pity or excessive sympathy is avoided. Good humor and laughter are an important aspect of any recreational program. Some features of a successful handicapped skiing organization are:

1. A financial base
2. Adaptive equipment
3. An equipment manager
4. Qualified instructors
5. A sympathetic ski area
6. Appropriate terrain and lifts

A strong financial base is necessary because skiing can be an expensive sport. A skier can easily spend $500 for the necessities of skis, boots, bindings, and a ski parka. Many disabled people do not have the financial resources to support a skiing hobby. Therefore, a successful handicapped skiing program provides equipment and lift tickets free to the disabled participant. A wide variety of equipment is necessary, including outrigger ski poles, skis of various sizes and models, boots, and specialized equipment such as the ski bra. A knowledgeable equipment manager also is critical to the club's operation, since equipment maintenance is a major factor in injury prevention.

One-on-one instruction lends optimal assistance to the new student who lacks confidence. Preferably a single instructor with a similar disability is paired with each student. Sometimes two instructors are assigned to a student if an able-bodied instructor is needed to help with lift lines or with falls. Such two-on-one instruction also helps new instructors gain familiarity with a wide variety of handicapping conditions and instructional techniques.

The teaching sequence for tri-track technique is as follows:

Walking

Falling

Getting up

Hop turn

Side step

Straight running

Stopping with outriggers

Riding the chair

Traverse

Uphill christy

Christy turn

Christy from a platform

Linked turns, shortswing

This sequence is essentially the same as that used in teaching able-bodied skiers, except that the wedge turn is eliminated from the tri-track technique. Tri-track skiing is loosely termed *monollel,* as opposed to the parallel skiing popular with two-ski enthusiasts. Turns are initiated with a gentle unweighting of the ski combined with a steering or torquing of the upper body. The rotational force transfers through the leg to the ski. Outriggers provide balance and assist in unweighting. Monollel is taught initially on flat terrain and then on very gentle open slopes. Repetition and practice is important.

Many disabled individuals need to spend additional time at home exercising to strengthen upper body, torso, and leg, because often they have not had opportunities to maintain fitness. Physical activity programs such as those offered by Gloria Stevens salons and Nautilus fitness centers and swimming programs can be joined by a disabled skier to help him or her achieve greater strength, flexibility, and cardiovascular fitness [2]. Individualized fitness programs can be prescribed by the physician, physical therapist, or occupational therapist.

A sympathetic ski area also is important to the success of any handicapped skiing program. Ski lift operators must be patient with individuals who need assistance in getting on or off the lifts. Negotiating lift lines is difficult for the amputee, who should be permitted ready access to the chair. Ski area administrators should be aware of the known risks involved for anyone who skis, whether able-bodied or disabled. Administrators should maintain good rapport with the director of the handicapped skiing school.

The risk of serious injury can be reduced if qualified instructors use individualized instruction for all participants, teach students how to fall safely, give lessons on appropriate terrain and snow conditions, and emphasize physical fitness and judgment during lessons.

Competition

Disabled people often have little opportunity to compete in sports activities; indeed, the greater the disability, the lesser is the opportunity. However, the drive to achieve and to compete is an aspect of human nature that cannot be ignored [3]. Whenever sports are engaged in, there is always the question of bettering one's previous performance: Can I score higher; lift more; ski faster? Whatever the sport, participants often entertain a strong desire to succeed.

Skiing can easily be a competitive sport. Slalom, giant slalom, and downhill racing are popular among many age groups and across many classes of skiers from novice to professional. National and international ski races are given extensive media coverage, thus further popularizing skiing as a competitive sport. Ski racing has become a regular facet of handicapped skiing clubs throughout the country. As of 1982, the National Handicapped Sports and Recreation Association had 32 chapters in 20 states. Regional handicapped skiing tournaments are held each year, and winners have an opportunity to compete in national and international championships. For these purposes, racers are classified according to their type of disability (Table 6-1).

Whether or not the disabled skier should race can ultimately be decided only by the skier. Many factors may influence this decision: Time commitment, personal interest, financial resources, peer pressure, parental interest, athletic talent, and competitive drive all play a role. The amputee is at special risk, which must also be considered.

Special Risks for Amputee Skiers

The chronic knee problem associated with chondromalacia is one of the most common limiting factors in the amputee skier whose one knee must do 100 percent of the work. The higher speeds and faster turns required in racing, combined with dry-land weight and fitness training, may rapidly accelerate degenerative joint pathology at the knee.

Many amputee skiers have required arthroscopy and joint surgery. Others have avoided knee problems through favorable biomechanics and anatomy, and still others have been able to prevent knee problems with the

Table 6-1
Classification of Disabled Skiers for Racing

Class	Disability or Body Part(s) Affected	Equipment Used
A-1	Both legs	Two regular-length skis and two outriggers
A-2	One leg	One regular-length ski and two outriggers or poles
A-3	Both legs	Two regular-length skis and two poles
A-4	One leg	Two regular-length skis and two poles
A-5, A-7	Both arms	Two regular-length skis and no poles
A-6, A-8	One arm	Two regular-length skis and one pole
A-9	One arm and one leg	Individual's choice
B-1	No sight	Guide
B-2	Vision of not more than 20/200 and/or visual field of ≤ 20 degrees with best optical correction	Guide

Note: Skiers with disabilities in more than two limbs have not yet been classified. These skiers should consult with the race committee at the time of the race.

frequent use of isometric quadriceps strengthening exercises. In general, knee stress can be reduced in the amputee skier if he or she skis in a more upright position, reduces the number of quick high-speed turns made, rests the thigh thoroughly between runs, avoids steep and mogul-ridden terrain, and avoids competitive situations when the knee is already sore.

Cold injury can be especially problematic for a disabled skier, since it is difficult for some disabled people to warm up properly. Before each run, the skier may warm up by hopping on the ski, swinging his or her arms back and forth, reclining on the ski and pushing the pelvis forward, embracing the knees in a crouch, and bending from side to side [4]. Stumps often are more susceptible to cold injury because of decreased circulation to the skin and subcutaneous tissues. Wool stump socks can be obtained, and a lightweight stump shell can be purchased from the prosthetist. This shell can be worn over the wool sock for added protection and insulation.

Instructors and assistants should watch for telltale signs of cold injury such as shivering or white frostbite patches on the cheeks. Instructors also should carry an extra pair of wool mittens for students with insufficient hand protection. Mittens rather than gloves should always be worn, especially by individuals using outriggers since pressure of the hands on the outriggers can decrease circulation in the fingers.

Lacerations of the face can occur when a student falls on outriggers. Early lessons teach the student to lift the outriggers up and away from the body during a fall. The Canadian crutch forearm band should be oriented with the opening away from the body to facilitate ease of removal in case of a fall.

Fatigue can be a major problem, especially for the beginning disabled skier. Some amputees will fatigue when standing for long periods of time on one leg. "Thigh burn" is a sign of excessive quadriceps strain in the amputee who makes long runs with accompanying knee flexion. Lying down for a moment's rest off the trail can relieve the muscles and give them time to recover. Other body areas, such as the neck, shoulders, and back, also can become tense. Progressive relaxation exercises performed beside the trail can relieve these tensions.

Everyone who skis has experienced the fear of falling, but amputees are used to falling; it is a part of their lives. Falling on snow is, in some ways, safer than falling on a hard floor. Physicians and other caregivers provide a valuable service in protecting handicapped individuals, but this can easily lead to overprotection. The disabled person finds it difficult to lead a complete life without the freedom to take some risks. An intelligent and balanced approach to sports participation can minimize risks and improve the quality of life for anyone.

References

1. Allen, A. *Sports for the Handicapped*. New York: Walker and Company, 1981.
2. Slusky, T.D. *The Skier's Year-Round Exercise Guide*. Briarcliff, N.Y.: Stein and Day, 1979.
3. Beaver, D.P., Jackson, R.W., McCann, B., et al. Roundtable: sport and recreation for the handicapped. *Physician Sportsmed.* 6:45–61, 1978.
4. Abraham, H. *Teaching Concepts: American Teaching Method*. Boulder, Colo.: Professional Ski Instructors of America, 1980, pp. 22–23.

III Psychological Considerations

7

Behavior Coaching: Some Practical Aspects in the New Health Psychology

Roger S. Zimmerman, Ph.D.

That how and where we lead our lives affects how healthy we are or are not may appear to be self-evident. Nonetheless, such knowledge is not uncomplicated. For example, *health* may be defined in a number of ways. Health may be considered the absence of disease, a definition that acknowledges what the phenomenon is not, rather than what it is. More inclusive definitions of health (e.g., an optimal level of biopsychosocial functioning) are more modernistic but may lack clinical or research usefulness. *How* and *where* imply choice, and choice is no more equally distributed than is opportunity. It can be argued that the unemployed have little choice, and that welfare mothers also have little choice, which is perhaps one of the reasons they rarely are among the ranks of joggers. The Kentucky coal miner may have chronic financial burdens matching his or her higher-than-average risk to chronic lung disease. Hence, his or her choices are limited, too. People whose health-related beliefs are rigidly defined, in effect, have limited choice as well.

Examination of the self-evident character of the relationship between health and life-style is useful. Choice involves options, and three factors affect the distribution of health-related options. These are (1) real options (or, more correctly, their absence); (2) the presence of a viable personal psychology (which consists of the ability to recognize, understand, develop, and act on real options); and (3) a sociocultural-political context that promotes and facilitates such recognition, understanding, development, and action. In brief, choice emerges from the interaction of perceived and dictated options, or the lack thereof.

There are a number of concerns and trends associated with this life-style/health options relationship. In this chapter, three of these trends are examined.

First, this relationship emphasizes that an individual's behavior plays a critical role in the determination of degrees of health or illness. The intricacies of this relationship—the mechanisms of action—have not always been clearly defined. Different methodologies, used by a variety of disciplines in typically less-than-perfect circumstances, have generated the data of interest to this health/life-style relationship. Although this relationship enjoys a long history, it has a short systematic past. Hence, one can expect some controversy regarding the findings, but one also can expect to find some useful guidance.

A second trend concerns behavioral science in general and psychology in particular. A strong interest in general health and behavior has developed among psychologists. Since the discipline of psychology focuses much of its energy on the study of behavior and since life-style broadly means behavioral patterns, it is not surprising that the role of health psychology in this area of health and behavior is growing.

Third, the current political climate[1] in the United States must be considered an important variable in the health/life-style relationship. This climate—conservative and atavistic—is consistent with the notion of individual responsibility and health. The term *life-style*, in fact, reflects the emphasis on responsibility and choice, and so it is not accidental that current political ideology in the United States has adopted this view. Politicians and ideologues often see only what they wish to see, and their vision may be blurred so that the distinction between responsibility and victim blaming becomes fuzzy.[2]

Individual Behavior as a Determinant of Health or Illness

Several recent publications and papers have reviewed the relationship between life-style, illness, and health [1–3]. Some life-style factors pertinent to this relationship are obesity, smoking, and poor stress management. Their relation to such phenomena as cardiovascular illness has been studied both retrospectively and prospectively [4]. The various so-called diseases of civilization—coronary artery disease, cerebrovascular illness, and some cancers (e.g., lung cancer)—account for nearly 70 percent of all deaths in the United States and an enormous amount of morbidity and disability [2].

Life-style factors involve behavioral patterns that are practiced repeatedly in a variety of stimulus situations. Some of these behaviors are displayed or emitted regularly (e.g., cigarette smoking) for a variety of reasons (e.g., perceived tension reduction) and the results are compromising to one's health. Some are not displayed in any regular fashion but have equally compromising effects (e.g., quieting [relaxation] responses). Zimmerman [5] summarized the relationship of life-style to health as follows:

> We are at higher risk (to illness) to the extent that we: eat too much, especially of saturated fats, smoke cigarettes, drink a lot of alcohol, remain

---

[1]This climate might best be described by the term *atavistic antigovernmentalism.*

[2]One consequence of the continuing (relative) lack of funding of preventive, educative, and health promotion programs is the continuation of victim blaming.

sedentary, drive too fast, live with great stress and little accompanying management of it, relate to others with buried hostility. . . .(p. 5)

A life filled with loneliness should be added to this list [6].

Others have characterized these life-style-related diseases as the "rusting-degenerative" disorders [7]. They include generalized arthero-sclerosis, essential hypertension, hyperlipemias, osteoporoses, chronic depression and anxiety states, chronic obstructive pulmonary disease, and the like. Increased risk to injuries due to overall poor physical fitness must also be included.

Although neither disease nor health is directly related to life-style, the relationships are not terribly convoluted either. Obesity provides a convenient example for looking at the links between these phenomena and also for reviewing some of the controversy surrounding the data. Eating too much and exercising too little typically results in an excess of input calories compared to output calories. Accumulation of fatty tissue and consequent weight gain follow. It is likely that genetically determined set-points, located in such subcortical brain areas as the hypothalamus, play a role in the dieting/weight loss/weight gain pattern that so often succeeds initial weight loss [8]. It remains to be seen exactly how influential these "weightostats" are in the overall determination of this pattern. It is generally believed that obesity places one at higher risk to a number of disorders, such as maturity-onset diabetes and some forms of coronary artery disease [9], but there is some controversy here as some investigators have suggested that obesity per se may not be an independent risk factor for cardiovascular disease [10].

Changing one's food intake response patterns and low caloric output patterns, according to the life-style perspective, would be the primary precursors to weight loss. Risk of coronary artery disease subsequently would drop. Changing these response patterns is, in effect, a life-style modification. A more complete change package would concern itself with cementing the changes. This cementing could be complicated and might require specialized helpers and change agents. For example, both group and individual counseling might prove helpful. Such counseling could focus on the meaning and symbolic value that food has for the individual, the role of early child-parent relations, development of reward patterns other than food rewards, and so forth.

Simple as the obesity example may make it sound, life-style modification is not easy. Furthermore, it is as difficult to be an effective facilitator of change as it is to be the person whose life-style is being modified. Among other things, change frequently means loss, and loss, even of undesirable behaviors, often has consequences for the individual's identity. The change agent does not cause a change in another's behavior so much as he or she facilitates the possibility of a change process. Thus, the change agent must proceed with awareness, knowledge of behavior, skills pertaining to methods of behavior change, and realistic goals. Some facets of the new health psychology may be helpful.

Health Psychology

Definition of Health Psychology

Psychology is concerned with behavior, but it also pays attention to thinking, feeling, motivation, personality development and functioning, social influence processes, mind-body relationships, and the like. Health psychology involves all the preceding concerns as they apply to problems of illness (e.g., the relationship of early child-parent interaction to a child's later development of gastrointestinal psychosomatic disorders) and of health (e.g., motivational conditions conducive to the acquisition of optimal health-related behaviors). Matarazzo [11] offers a more comprehensive definition of health psychology:

> Health psychology is the aggregate of the specific educational, scientific, and professional contributions of the discipline of psychology to the promotion and maintenance of health, the prevention and treatment of illness, and the identification of etiologic and diagnostic correlates of health, illness, and related dysfunction. . . .(p. 815)

Health psychology is a broad term which encompasses such older subspecialties as medical psychology and such newer subspecialties as behavioral medicine and behavioral health. These latter areas are strongly interdisciplinary in character and are concerned with the various shades of gray between medicine, behavioral science, clinical psychology, and psychosomatics. Some other relevant areas include public health, medical sociology, applied social psychology, anthropology, and medical economics. Public education may also be relevant—for example, in planning a mass media campaign aimed at preventing the development of beliefs congruent with cigarette smoking in elementary-school-aged children [12].

If, as has been postulated, *life-style* broadly means behavioral patterns, and if such patterns are related to disease and health, then psychology in general, and health psychology in particular, will play a major role in our understanding of health- and illness-related behaviors. Such understanding is likely to be helpful—perhaps even critical—in the design of programs that ultimately concern behavioral change. There is some evidence that the frequency and intensity of life-style behaviors that affect health and illness can be altered, and risk reduction is a likely consequence [13]. Knowles [2], a physician, suggested, ". . . control of the present major health problems in the U.S. depends directly on modification of the individual's behavior and habits of learning" (p. 61).

Behavioral interventions frequently find their theoretical origin in activities that have preceded the development of health psychology. Although health psychology is a recent development, behavior modification is a good decade or two older. There is well-established behavior modification research and a large body of clinically oriented literature, some of which is of interest to the health psychologist. Some examples are modification of verbal behavior associated with coronary-prone (type A) behavior, contingency management and medication compliance, and operant strategies for reducing dropout rates in exercise programs. Other change agents and health professionals, such as family practitioners, might share an interest in some of these areas.

Behavior Coaching

The concept of behavior coaching finds its origin in the blend of health psychology and behavior modification. Alterations of behavior often will take the form of either increases or decreases in frequency or intensity. There are some general principles of behavior coaching, which will be reviewed later in this chapter, but it is important to discuss first the general notion of behavior coaching.

A behavior coach is a person who is likely to play multiple roles in his or her primary job or job setting. This person might be a psychologist, a family practitioner, a pediatric nurse practitioner (working with a mother), or a dentist. This person might also be working (working with a mother), or a or another: For example, he or she may be a nurse's aid who works in a nursing home. The major role of a behavior coach is to help another person (client, patient, or student) help himself or herself alter behavior, specifically health- or illness-related behaviors.

Behavior coaches have certain things in common with other good coaches.[3] Athletic coaches do not win games; the team wins the game and the good coach will have helped in that process. Likewise, in the world of behavior coaching, winning means helping a client or patient move in the direction of health, in the direction of higher levels of biologic and psychosocial functioning, thereby decreasing that person's risk to the rusting-degenerative disorders, the sequelae of disuse and misuse.

People who function as behavior coaches must understand something about motivation both as a process and as a set of principles [14]. They may have some formal educational experience in this area or an almost intuitive

---

[3]For some people, the term *coach* has unfortunate associations. "Out of control" or "winning is all" may come to mind. My use of this term is as a reasonably accurate descriptor of what we might do with clients or patients: Just as athletic coaches are charged with the responsibility of helping athletes attain optimal athletic performance, behavior coaches must help their clients achieve their optimal behavioral health potential.

grasp of the essentials of this process, and they are able to apply the principles in effective ways. They also must understand the social psychology of influence and persuasion. They have a sense of when to remain at ease and when to exert pressure. They know that change and development take time. A sense of humor is required.

It follows from the preceding description that behavior coaches, drawn from other disciplines and other roles, play a variety of subroles and serve multiple functions. They are educators, instructors, exhorters, directors, teachers, and suggesters. The best of them appear to be able to balance and blend a measure of authoritativeness with adherence to democratic principles of decision making. This blend promotes the possibility of partnership between the coach and the individual being coached, so the latter is more likely to become actively invested in and committed to the change process. As a result, the potential for reducing risk to illness, on the one hand, and for attaining optimal health, on the other hand, probably will take explicit form.

Change does not emanate directly from the coach, and it does not emanate directly from the quality of the coach-client relationship. Excellent rapport probably is a necessary condition for change to occur—it constitutes a facilitative mechanism—but, in and of itself, such rapport is not a sufficient condition to effect change. The relationship between coach and client must be reasonably intense, reasonably personal, and have elements of mutual feedback, but such a relationship also may involve counterproductive elements of overdependency.

The behavior coach often must enlist various elements of the client's or patient's social system and support network. Where no such network exists, the coaching role will include exercises, prompts, and plays to help the coached individual develop such a network, because change needs support, and specifically, social support. The coach must understand the general principles of such systems and such support as well as something about the particular client's unique social system. The major problem in behavior change is not initiation but maintenance, and maintenance of change is more likely to the extent that one's immediate social context supports such change. For example, psychotherapy with the married alcoholic is unlikely to succeed in the absence of therapeutic work with the spouse as well. Dropout rates from exercise programs, which can run as high as 50 percent or more, provides another example. The participant is likely to drop out if he or she has feelings of isolation from everyone else. Such feelings become further entrenched with a presumed continued deficit in social and interactional skills. Behavior coaches must be knowledgeable about teaching such skills. They also must be informed about community resources, including the means for increasing the client's contacts with his or her natural social system. In fact, the behavior coach often may function less as a coach on an individual basis than as a behavioral engineer consultant in terms of promoting systems changes.

Behavior Coaching as Intervention

Pogo—not Freud—was the greatest twentieth-century psychologist, for he said, "We have met the enemy and he is us." To paraphrase Pogo's declaration, people generally end up doing what they want to do, our efforts to the contrary notwithstanding. Despite the truth of this statement, we remain optimistic, even if dourly so. It is difficult, but not impossible, to make people stop engaging in illness-related behaviors and start practicing optimal health behaviors.

There are three critical categories of practical aspects of the new health psychology: general principles of behavior-coached programs, data gathering, and strategic interventions. Let us look first at the general principles.

General Principles. The following list provides some general principles of behavior-coached programs:

Awareness (knowledge)

Relationship building
    Patience and developing rapport
    Empathic listening; communication skills
    Flexibility
    Active involvement; creating the partnership

The change process
    Change and identity
    Change process characteristics
    What to change
    How to initiate change: Feedback and reinforcement
    How to maintain change: Relapse as a process
    Realistic goal setting
    Importance of the social context: Microenvironments and
    macroenvironments

Emphasis of the positive aspects of the change process
    Positive expectations
    Avoidance of being judgmental
    Slip-ups and discussions of fear of failure
    Using the placebo effect

Follow-up
    Cementing the changes
    Side effects (overdependency)

Avoiding coach burn-out
    Critical questions
    Consultations with others
    Pogo's dictum
    Has the program worked (without your seeing it)?

As this list implies, patient awareness is the foundation of any behavior-coached program. The patient or client already has a modicum of awareness—that is, he or she knows that something is not as it should be. Behavior coaches build on this awareness by employing appropriate teaching and communication skills. Clients are approached as potential partners in a health-building enterprise in which patience and flexibility are the bricks and mortar. Active involvement facilitates the learning that provides the bedrock for change.

Coaches must listen carefully. Those who lack requisite empathic listening skills are themselves in need of coaching to acquire these skills. Questions such a coach should ask himself or herself include: Should I be working with this person? Should I refer my client elsewhere? Do I need a consultant?

The change process tends to be slow, continuous, and incremental. A behavior coach must be cautious about sudden major changes. Alternatively, he or she must be open to displays of insight and their potential healing quality. In any case, the change process should not be rushed. Exhortations may work on occasion, but they also may boomerang, yielding such unintended side effects as arousal of unresolved, adolescentlike authority conflicts.

Willpower and the lack of it have been discussed for years, usually to no avail. In behavior coaching, the focus is more appropriately the will to prepare. Such an emphasis will direct the coach and the client to be concerned with the conditions under which a behavior occurs and the conditions under which it is likely to change. To discover these conditions, coaches may have to push and pull their clients, but they will learn to modify their behavior in this regard. People often proceed at a pace that is consistent with their needs. Coaches are aware of the inherent mutuality of their relationship with the people they coach. A true applied psychology of persuasion recognizes that feedback is a two-way proposition.

Working together, the coach and client will decide (1) what to change, (2) how best to initiate the change, and (3) how best to maintain the change. A working partnership is likely to yield a set of realistic goals.

Reinforcement and feedback regarding knowledge of the results is critical. The client or patient should be educated about the importance of reinforcement in learning and behavior change. The rewards and benefits of life-style change—more energy, feeling better, higher productivity, and the like—should be emphasized.

Behavior coaches must be knowledgeable about reinforcement as a process and reinforcers as events (see pp. 84 and 85). Each should ask himself or herself: Do I need coaching? Am I working with my local behavior modifier? Have I seen videotapes of myself dispensing social reinforcement? Could I be more effective in this regard?

The behavior coach should emphasize the positive aspects of behavior changing and should avoid being judgmental. Slip-ups should be expected, since the initiation of behavior change is much less of a problem than the maintenance of such change. For the given behavior in question, it is helpful to determine whether there is a relapse path which has potential intervention points. Negative expectations must not be communicated to the client. Open, frank discussion of such common maladies as fear of failure often is helpful.

As in other professions, burn-out appears to be an occupational hazard of behavior coaching. It must be remembered that this task involves a partnership between the coach and the client. With realistic goals, the partnership can at least move in the right direction, which is better than not moving at all.

Data Gathering. The essentials of data gathering for a behavior-coached program can be summarized as follows:

General impressions
  Style of relating
  Issues of self-esteem
  Brief mental status screen; premorbid adjustment

Traditional data base
  Biographic data
  Biopsychosocial indicants
  Significant medical history
  Significant psychosocial history

Health-related behaviors checklist
  Substance use and abuse
  Exercise (aerobics)
  Diet and nutritional status (weight)
  Coronary-prone behavior: Modified Jenkins type A questionnaire

Stress managment
Thinking style (e.g., rigid versus flexible)
Emotional style (e.g., denier, accepter, or expresser)
Quality of interpersonal relationships
Social contexts
Loneliness

Behavior analysis
Target behavior
Joint decision making and realistic goal setting
Using behavior logs and self-assessment scales
Conditions analysis
Behavior flow
Antecedents
Consequences
Behavior history
Duration of target behavior
Variations in frequency and intensity
Past change attempts
Preferred reinforcers

The coach must first catalog his or her overall general impression of the client or patient. (For instance, is he or she a hurried executive or a passive or aggressive skilled worker?) How the coach forms these impressions also is important, since self-knowledge, or its lack, can affect the coaching process in a variety of ways.

The client's style of relating to the coach requires assessment. Is it characteristic of that person's relating style? Some people are more comfortable in authoritative relationships, whereas others prefer strictly democratic decision making. Many people probably respond best to some balance between these two poles. In fact, it is most likely that relating styles will vary at different stages in the behavioral change process. That is, at the stage of behavioral change initiation, some measure of authoritativeness may be best, whereas an emphasis on democratic decision making may prove to be most effective during the latter stages of change maintenance.

The initial assessment, impression formation, and determination of the client's style of relating are inextricable from the client's sense of self-confidence. What role is this variable playing in the client's life? Coaches often can obtain an intuitive fix on this issue of self-esteem.

It is important to obtain a fair amount of detail regarding such traditional data as the client's occupational status, living situation, family life, marital status, and life satisfactions. Information pertaining to the client's personal medical history, as well as his or her family's medical history, also is important and may influence recommendations regarding behavior changes. The potential influence of medical histories on a behavioral change program has been discussed at length elsewhere [7]. Working relationships with physicians and nurse practitioners are essential. One should not assume that assessment of risk factors on the behavioral level alone is adequate.

A psychosocial history is critical. The coach should have either training in collecting psychosocial data or a means of collecting, understanding, and evaluating this data via relationships with other aids. The history should include a good sketch of how the person carries on his or her psychological business with the world.

As indicated in the list of data gathering essentials (p. 81–82), the checklist includes such variables as thinking style and emotional style. These variables play important roles in health and illness. They also play significant roles in the application of intervention strategies. Coronary-prone behavior frequently can be evaluated using questionnaires and careful observation, as in structured interviewing. Other resources and forms that may prove useful in helping clients manage stress better can be found in Jenny Steinmetz, Jon Blankenship, Linda Brown, et al., *Managing Stress Before it Manages You* (Palo Alto: Bull Publishing Co., 1980).

The behavior analysis probably is the most important part of data gathering for behavior coaching. There are three critical parts.

First, the *target behavior* must be identified and the direction of intended change (e.g., increase or decrease) must be specified. Will the change be one in frequency (e.g., less smoking) or intensity (e.g., more intense aerobic exercise)? The client's use of behavior diaries or logs is necessary to obtain baseline data to facilitate setting realistic goals. The frequency, amount, time of day, and, if relevant, feelings associated with a certain behavior should be recorded. Feelings can be evaluated on a three-point scale—mild, moderate, or severe.

The second critical part of behavior analysis is *conditions analysis.* That is, under what conditions does the behavior occur, and under what conditions is it maintained? These conditions include antecedent (stimulus) ones (such as anxiety prior to reaching for a cigarette) and consequent (reinforcement) one (such as displaying type A behavior [e.g., hostility, impatience] to avoid interactions with other people, which engender anxiety).

Third, a behavior history must be obtained. Questions that should be answered include: How long-lasting is the behavior in question? Furthermore, when did it develop, does it have a natural history, and does it ebb and flow seemingly apart from changes in environmental conditions? If there were attempts to change it in the past, to what degree were they successful? What type of behavior is it? (For instance, there are six factors that characterize cigarette smoking behavior. If one or two factors predominate for a particular smoker, then he or she is that type.)

Data gathering is an important task, and therefore it should be done slowly and carefully. The assessment and classification of types of behavior have treatment implications. For example, the habitual smoker frequently responds to approaches to which the "crutch" smoker does not respond. A good behavioral analysis may take 1 to 3 hours. Helpers must budget their time accordingly and be able to use inventories and questionnaires in an efficient manner.

Strategic Interventions. The following list summarizes the major factors in strategic intervention:

Role model (asking tough questions of oneself)

Behavioral change initiation
    Program and target behavior review
    Behavior recording forms
    Shaping (successive approximation): Response display
    Reinforcement
        Response probability
        Frequency and intensity
        Immediacy and repetition
        Making the transition to self-control procedures
    Approach-avoidance analysis
    Procedural examples
        Relaxation training
    Thought stopping

Behavioral change maintenance
    The relapse path
        Discussions of the psychology of persistence
        Strengthening new behavior bonds
    Assessment and analysis: Behavioral monitoring
    Treatment recommendations
        Review of program rationale
        Time management
          Goal setting
          Prioritization
        Role playing
        Telephone contact
        Using significant others
    Procedural examples
        Contingency contracting
        Renegotiation of contracts
        Imagery training

Social contexts
Follow-up
  Expectations
  Discussions
Consultations with local behavior modifiers

The coach's presentation of himself or herself as an appropriate role model is critical to the success of a behavior-coached program. Stressed, smoking, overweight coaches are not likely to inspire their clients to modify their behaviors. Each coach must ask himself or herself hard questions pertaining to his or her own life, questions about emotional stability, balance between work and play, and balance in thinking style between flexibility and authoritativeness. Also important are questions pertaining to the practice of health-related behaviors in the coach's own life.

As has been indicated previously, helping a person initiate behavior change generally is less of a problem than maintaining that change. Initiation factors include target behavior review, appropriate design and use of behavior recording forms, review of goals, and the importance of new response display. Important principles here include the concept of shaping or successive approximation, by which small components of the overall behavior are reinforced as long as they represent movement in the right direction. A thorough discussion of how the client will carry on such reinforcement on his or her own is likely to be more productive than one focusing on vague and nebulous notions of self-control, discipline, and the like.

Do all parties concerned understand the concept of reinforcement and its intricacies? Does the coach need coaching? Behavior (response patterns) tends to be elicited under the influence of antecedent stimulus conditions; it tends to be controlled by immediate consequences. Careful behavior analysis is necessary to distinguish these variables (see the list of data gathering elements, pp. 81–82). Reinforcement refers to response probability, and a reinforcer is an event that increases response strength (frequency and intensity) in that it increases the likelihood of response occurrence in the future. To make reinforcement more meaningful for the client or patient, the coach needs those communication skills that are flexible enough to facilitate giving helpful explanations.

Some behaviors are strengthened by approach (positive) reinforcers. For example, smoking probability increases as a function of perceived tension reduction. Other behaviors are strengthened by avoidance (negative) reinforcers. For instance, smoking probability increases as a function of avoiding or mitigating unpleasant withdrawal symptoms. An approach-avoidance analysis is an important assessment tool that also constitutes a type of strategic intervention. As with the cigarette smoking example, the initiation of most behaviors is associated with a predominance of one or the other sets of reinforcement conditions, but the maintenance of behaviors generally involves the interaction of both sets of conditions.

Punishment refers to procedures designed to weaken behavior. Such procedures may sometimes be helpful (such as increasing the costs of membership in an exercise program as the percent of dropouts increases), but the effects tend to be transient. Punishment tends to suppress behavior rather than weaken it. Such procedures also may create the occasion for unresolved authority conflicts to surface. Issues pertaining to fear of failure (and success) also may surface as a consequence of punishment. The quality of rapport may suffer, and the coach's own feelings may get in the way of providing effective intervention. It must be remembered that people tend to respond in terms of their beliefs and perceptions, which are at least as influential as objective reality.

Maintaining behavior change means reducing the likelihood of relapse [15]. Both the coach and client will benefit from a discussion of the psychology of persistence. Role playing often is helpful as part of the preparation for encountering situations associated with a high probability of relapse. For example, how does the subassertive alcoholic learn to say "no" with minimal feelings of guilt when confronted with the opportunity to drink in the local bar which happens to be his or her only effective social outlet? Some of the variables important to the enhancement of compliance with health-related programs include a review of the program rationale, time management procedures, continued contact between the coach and client, renegotiation of primary and contingency agreements, and the use of significant others in the client's life to aid in monitoring the client's overall behavior. In addition, it may prove valuable for the coach to encourage the client to telephone him or her when particular problems arise, when advice or support is needed, and so on.

Scheduled follow-up visits are important. Reassessment of some problem areas may occur during these visits, and they provide an opportunity to monitor and reinforce behaviors as appropriate. The kind of progress being made can be determined, and the likelihood of relapse can be evaluated: Is this likelihood declining or at least stabilizing? Follow-up visits also allow the coach and client to determine whether either party's expectations have changed. A client's feelings of failure may have to be defused to minimize other negative feelings such as those associated with diminished self-efficacy. During these visits, the coach must remain acutely aware of all aspects of the communication process, since nonverbal communications can have powerful effects on clients.

Once a relatively firm change in behavior has taken place, it takes on a kind of flywheel quality. That is, it seemingly runs by itself. There usually is a reduced need for the continuation of behavior monitoring forms and some of the other emphases characteristic of the initiation phase. The coach and client can work together in making decisions in this area through a partnership format.

Behavior Prescription. In this section, the outline of a behavior prescription based on work with a hypothetical client is presented. It actually is a kind of composite picture drawn from past or ongoing behavior coaching.

The client is a 44-year-old married carpenter who also works occasionally as a realtor. The significant medical history includes mild adult-onset diabetes and "tennis elbow." On a stress electrocardiogram test he showed definite signs of fatigue during mild to moderate levels of aerobic work. He appears to be approximately 10 to 20 lb overweight.

He presented initially with some mild depression and anxiety. This was related both to the beginnings of some marital difficulty (his second marriage) and some loss of interest in carpentry. The latter, it was discovered, was connected to a decline in the client's physical energy over the past several years. Although in interview situations he related in an adequate manner, he was not especially warm or spontaneous. He was somewhat introspective, which was advantageous to realistic goal setting and in his initial acceptance of the referral from a family practitioner.

Table 7-1 shows the behavior prescription assigned to this patient. The recommendations in the behavior prescription were followed initially with some enthusiasm. However, the marital difficulties continued, and as they did, interest in and compliance with recommendations declined. Following the behavior coach's suggestion for marriage counseling, which was successful, the client's maintenance of behavioral change improved.

The coaching program, including the marriage counseling, took approximately 4 months of weekly visits followed by 2 months of bimonthly visits. The client also enrolled in a community education stress management course.

Larger Considerations: Contexts and Change

Microsocial Contexts

As was mentioned earlier, change does not emanate directly from the quality of the coach-client relationship. Rather, change emanates directly from the individual for a variety of reasons under a variety of conditions. One such condition is the good helping relationship, characterized by understanding, mutuality, acceptance, and genuineness. If the coached person is fairly coachable, the chances for successful behavioral change are even better.

It is necessary, too, to extend the behavioral change program beyond the coach-client relationship. People carry out their psychological business with the world in multiple, largely social contexts. Therefore, maintenance of change is more likely to occur when the client's immediate social system, such

Table 7-1
Behavior Prescription

Diet and nutrition
1. Reduce overall salt and sugar intake
2. Reduce saturated fat intake by approximately 10%
3. Increase fiber intake by approximately 10-20%
   a. Nutritionist's approval
   b. Menu lists
4. Weight: To be reconsidered in 3 mo; also consider contingency contracting re enrollment
            in local diet center

Substance use and abuse
1. Nonproblematic
2. Spouse is smoker: 1 pack daily for 10-15 yr; smoked low-tar cigarettes for last 2 yr
   a. Discuss tactful tactics to discourage spouse's behavior
   b. Take home literature

Aerobic exercise
1. Electrocardiogram stress test clearance
2. Take home literature
3. Names and telephone numbers of contact people, local aerobics program; consider integrating into practice group of runners in 3 mo
4. Fitness discussion
   a. F.I.T.[a] formula
   b. Night running safety

Stress management
1. Discussion of "bibliotherapy"
2. Names and telephone numbers of contact people about community education stress management program
3. Relaxation tape; imagery book

Personal
1. Marriage counseling (referral?)
2. Discussion re negative self-messages (assertive training course?)

Other: Balance between work and play

[a]F = frequency of aerobic exercise (3 times a week); I = intensity at 75% of maximum heart rate; T = time or duration of each workout (20-30 min).

as spouse and friends, is supportive. It may be equally important to involve larger sociocultural systems, such as the work place, union, and civic organizations. These systems can be influenced to support health-related behavioral changes on the part of individuals. In such cases, coaches may have to function as a kind of behavioral engineer, able to conduct consultations with components of the social system. Such consultations may include discussions of incentive rearrangements, factors that enhance productivity, and the like.

Another variable that sometimes affects how long-lasting change is concerns the impact of the change on other people. Not everyone may like the client's new behavior patterns. Weight loss provides an example. There are some marital relationships in which the always-thin spouse may have a psychological stake in keeping the other spouse overweight. Such stakes and claims may outlast behavior changes. Adherence to schedules of increased caloric output can crumble in the face of sophisticated (and often unconscious) sabotage strategies. Again, coaches must realize that clients or patients do not live in a vacuum. Behavior tends to be a social affair.

Macrosocial Contexts

Larger, macrosocial contexts also affect behavior change. Health care policy is carved from the politics, ideology, and economics of this larger social system. It is doubtful that the results of behavioral science research contribute very much to the development of this policy. So what views does the macrosocial context promulgate about prevention of illness and promotion of health?

Some people argue that the major problem with the health care system in the United States is that it is nonexistent as such and that what we have is an illness care complaint-response system. The government has paid lip service to prevention efforts but has not funded such efforts. Former President Carter, in 1978, said:

> We have spent 40 cents out of every health dollar on hospitalization. In effect, we've made the hospital the first line of defense instead of the last. By contrast, we've spent only 3 cents on disease prevention and control, less than ½ cent on health education, and ¼ cent on environmental health research.

Many consequences follow from this policy, including increased power of traditional hospital lobby groups, collusion between the medical technical industry and these lobby groups, and perpetuation of the notion that medical care and proximity to hospitals are primary determinants of health. Another consequence is that, generally speaking, modification of health-related behaviors is not a reimbursable service. Contemporary knowledge derived from behavioral psychology suggests that incentives are powerful regulators and encouragers of behavior. Incentives must exist, be in place, and be operational if we expect to develop firm institutional supports for a rational prevention-oriented, health promotion, health care system.

As Taylor [16] has pointed out, "Increasingly, preventive strategies are being shaped by an ideology that attributes to individuals the responsibility for their own health and well-being. . ." (p. 1). The politics of prevention must be addressed if the psychology and biology of this enterprise are to have any basis in reality. It is not at all surprising, then, that the current Reagan administration ideology and the emphasis on individual responsibility are complementary. Such an emphasis is almost wholly one-sided. The current trend in political ideology has spawned policies that inhibit the development and growth of modern, broadly defined public health programs. As a result, a variety of social and educational programs are not seen as an intrinsic part of public health policy. Instead, such programs are viewed as unnecessary politically liberal appendages. Individual responsibility has become an ideologic banner with marked implications for conceptualization and programming in public health. A good example of this is the recent dismantling, via radical budget cuts, of the environmental regulatory apparatus. What has emerged is a type of "social law": there is an inverse relationship between emphasis on individual responsibility and deemphasis on eliminating industrial pollution, as far as health maintenance is concerned. Of related interest are the ways in which the so-called holistic health movement adds to the overemphasis on the model of individual responsibility.

That the current administration may be too inspired by the legions of the "worried well" who are jogging, managing stress, and losing weight is a real concern. In the meantime, the large-scale problem called *acid rain* is said to require more study, chemical dump contents infiltrate our aquifers, and tobacco subsidies continue, despite the surgeon general's warning (albeit restrained) of the consequences to health of cigarette smoking behavior. There may be aspects of the new health psychology, including our notions of behavior coaching, that either fit or can easily be made to fit this lopsided individual behavior model. An area awaiting more definitive theoretical development is the formulation of public health policy wedded to good principles of behavior modification.

What is needed is a balance between a social approach and an individual approach to health care and health promotion [17]. The value of such a balance would take into account, in terms of systems development, such things as environmental threats to health and behavioral technology that can help people deal with ongoing problems now. Ideologic positions that can find only profit motivation behind corporate concern with worker health are rigid, as are narrow individualist interpretations of illness prevention. We must find some balance because accommodation is likely to yield a political reality consistent with the development of a rational health care system.

Early in this chapter, we discussed choice and options. A sociopolitical context that offers some of the balance just alluded to is more likely to offer realistic options to larger numbers of people. It also would promote the recognition of these options and encourage action and behavior consistent with them. One consequence would be that the line between individual responsibility and victim blaming would become more distinct (see p. 74).

A Fourth Trend

Thus far, we have discussed three trends associated with the health/life-style relationship, but there is a fourth trend that also deserves mention. It is concerned with the trendiness of trends. That medicine and behavioral science influence the culture in which they exist is obvious. This is, perhaps, one of the distinguishing characteristics of our age. However, that the reverse is likely to be true is less obvious.

Are we suddenly in danger of being inundated by holistic waves of new programs? What will happen when the newness effect wears off? There are three recent cultural forces that have impacted on the culture-health-behavior matrix. These forces are the narcissistic excesses of the 1970s, the reemergence of antiintellectualism, and the development of new marketing strategies for selling "old snake oil." The most unfortunate aspect of this probably is the Jacobin-like reaction that may develop. Recently, excessive reaction often takes the form of throwing the baby out with the bath water.

Recently there have been some important new developments regarding health-related behaviors (e.g., increased understanding of the biochemistry of the placebo effect). What makes these developments so important and so exciting is, in part, that their time indeed has come. Perhaps the time also has arrived for the development of a health-care system that (1) is oriented toward genuine health care, (2) provides for the pivotal role of the behavior coach, and (3) is socially and politically responsive to the public health demands of the 1980s.

References

1. Engels, G.L. The need for a new medical model: a challenge for biomedicine. *Science* 196:129–136, 1977.

2. Knowles, J.H. (ed.). *Doing Better and Feeling Worse.* New York: Norton, 1977.

3. LaLonde, M.A. *A New Perspective on the Health of Canadians.* Ottawa, Canada: Ministry of National Health and Welfare Information, 1975.

4. Paffenbarger, R.S., Wing, A.L., Hyde, R.T. Physical activity and an index of heart attack risk in college alumni. *Am. J. Epidemiol.* 108:161–175, 1978.

5. Zimmerman, R.S. Health: Attainment, Maintenance, and Optimization—The Psychologist as Behavior Coach (abstract). Paper presented at the Max Planck Institute for Psychiatry, Munich, West Germany, January 1981. *Am. J. Prev.* In press.

6. Lynch, J. *The Broken Heart: Medical Consequences of Loneliness.* New York: Basic Books, 1979.

7. Childs, H.D. Exercise and life-style modification in family practice. In Cantu, R.C. (ed.), *Health Maintenance Through Physical Conditioning.* Littleton, Mass.: PSG Publishing, 1981.

    8. Stunkard, A.J.   Why Obesity Looks Like an Addiction. Paper presented at the Conference on Addictive Behaviors, Harvard Medical School, Boston, October 1982.
    9. Stamler, J.   The primary prevention of coronary heart disease. In Baunwalde, E. (ed.), *The Myocardium: Failure and Infarction.* New York: H.P. Publishing, 1974.
    10. Agras, W.S.   Weight reduction and blood pressure management: the generalized and enduring effects of two behavior change procedures. In Stuart, R.B. (ed.), *Adherence, Compliance, and Generalization in Behavioral Medicine.* New York: Brunner/Mazel, 1982.
    11. Matarazzo, J.D.   Behavioral health and behavioral medicine: frontiers for a new health psychology. *Am. Psychol.* 35:807–817, 1980.
    12. Evans, R.I.   Research in the social psychology of persuasion and behavior modification: relevant to school health education? *J. Sch. Health* 13(2):110–113, 1973.
    13. Stuart, R.B. (ed.).   *Adherence, Compliance, and Generalization in Behavioral Medicine.* New York: Brunner/Mazel, 1982.
    14. Wilt, F., Bosen, K.   *Motivation and Coaching Psychology.* Los Altos, Calif.: Tafnews Press, 1971.
    15. Marlatt, G.A., Gordon, J.R.   Determinants of relapse: implications for the maintenance of behavior change. In Davidson, P.O., Davidson, S.M. (eds.), *Behavioral Medicine: Changing Health Lifestyles.* New York: Brunner/Mazel, 1980.
    16. Taylor, R.   The politics of prevention. *Soc. Policy.* In press.
    17. Venkateson, M.   Preventive health care and marketing: positive aspects. In Cooper, P.D., Kehoe, W.J., Murphy, P.E. (eds.), *Marketing and Preventive Health Care: Interdisciplinary and Interorganizational Perspectives.* Chicago: American Marketing Association, 1978.

8 Using Perceived Exertion for the Prescription of Exercise in Healthy Adults

Edmund J. Burke, Ph.D.
Marcia L. Collins, M.S.

A basic principle of exercise physiology is that a systematic prudent exercise program over time will result in a series of apparently beneficial physiologic alterations in the body, collectively referred to as the *training effect* [1–3]. Understanding the role of oxygen may help us determine what a *prudent* program is.

The Fick equation ($\dot{V}o_2 = \dot{Q}t \times [Cao_2 - C\bar{v}o_2]$ tells us that oxygen consumption per minute ($\dot{V}o_2$) is equal to the product of cardiac output ($\dot{Q}t$) and the arteriovenous oxygen content difference. ($Cao_2 - C\bar{v}o_2$ *or* $C[a\text{-}\bar{v}]o_2$). In simple terms, oxygen consumption is a function of the amount of oxygenated blood pumped and the ability of the muscle cell to take up and use the oxygen from the arterial blood. Over time, the continuous transport of oxygen, first by the lungs and subsequently by the circulatory system, and eventually the actual oxygen uptake at the muscle cell site seems to result in the training effect. Just how the transport and uptake of oxygen causes the training effect is still a matter of active investigation, but several possible mechanisms are that:

Diffusion of gases across the alveolar membrane is increased.

Saturation and desaturation of hemoglobin in red blood cells is increased.

There is increased contraction of heart muscle against greater resistance (more blood and increased arterial pressure).

Blood vessels may alter due to hypoxia or the increased blood volume.

Mitochondria appear to respond to increased O_2 uptake by increasing in size and number.

Thus, it should be clear that *oxygen is the key to the training effect*. Exercise-induced increases in $\dot{V}o_2$ clearly are important, but it must be realized that an appropriate $\dot{V}o_2$ level for one individual might have little effect in eliciting a training effect in a second individual and could cause grave health hazards to a third person. Exercise $\dot{V}o_2$ must be individualized.

Everyone has a maximal level of oxygen consumption per unit of time ($\dot{V}_{O_2}$ max) which has been influenced by heredity and his or her life-style (i.e., the level of exercise-induced $\dot{V}_{O_2}$). To put it in terms of the Fick equation, every person's ability to pump and move blood and to use the O_2 from the arterial blood is limited. To test one's $\dot{V}_{O_2}$ max, the individual is asked to increase gradually some type of work until he or she reaches the level at which an increasing workload elicits no further increase in $\dot{V}_{O_2}$. As the workload ($\dot{V}_{O_2}$) is increased, the work becomes more difficult. This is primarily because with each increasing workload, more and more of the metabolic waste product lactic acid is being produced. At some point, the level of lactic acid is associated with a nonlinear rise in ventilation. As described by Wasserman et al. [4], this point is referred to as the *anaerobic threshold*. Since oxygen consumption is the key to the training effect, it follows that the higher the person's anaerobic threshold is—that is, the higher the percentage of $\dot{V}_{O_2}$ max at which the individual can work—without undue fatigue, the closer the training effect will come to being the maximal attainable for that individual.

The American College of Sports Medicine (ACSM) [5] has reviewed the scientific literature and established guidelines for exercise prescription (i.e., they have attempted to answer our question about what is prudent). The ACSM has recommended that individuals exercise at least three times per week, each exercise period lasting at least 1 hour, with the exercise period divided into a warm-up, a stimulus, and a cool-down phase. During the stimulus phase, which is the part of the exercise period most responsible for eliciting the training effect, the ACSM recommends that the individual work at between 50 and 85 percent of his or her $\dot{V}_{O_2}$ max, but short of measuring oxygen, which is very costly, how do we know when we are working at a given percentage of our $\dot{V}_{O_2}$ max?

Heart Rate as a Predictor of Percent Maximal Oxygen Consumption

For the last two decades, heart rate has been the most common means of individualizing an exercise program. It has been the most common means of assessing the percentage of $\dot{V}_{O_2}$ max elicited during exercise. Indeed, the ACSM [5] has recommended that the stimulus portion of the exercise period be performed at 60 to 90 percent of maximal heart rate reserve. It must be remembered, however, that heart rate is being used as a predictor of the percentage of $\dot{V}_{O_2}$ max, not as an end in itself. Let us examine the advantages and limitations of heart rate as such a predictor.

Advantages

Heart rate assessment is fairly easy to teach to a novice. Immediately following exercise, the exerciser can palpate either the radial or carotid artery and, within a few sessions, can become fairly proficient at measuring his or her true heart rate [6,7]. Adding this scientific element to an exercise program also may improve motivation, since an individual can obtain immediate feedback about the physical benefits (e.g., lowered exercise heart rate) of the program.

Heart rate may be correlated with electrocardiographic arrhythmias or other abnormalities related to coronary artery disease, such as angina, during a stress test. The exerciser then is cautioned to exercise at a safe level below the heart rate that was associated with abnormalities.

Heart rate usually is linearly related to $\dot{V}O_2$. It is well known that heart rate increases with increased work and increased $\dot{V}O_2$ [8].

Disadvantages

The use of heart rate as a predictor of percent $\dot{V}O_2$ max also has limitations. Although heart rate assessment is fairly easy to learn, the exerciser most likely to make heart rate assessment errors is the novice, who most needs to work at a safe level. In addition, heart rate is affected by environmental factors such as temperature and emotional factors such as nervousness. This tends to decrease the relationship between heart rate and $\dot{V}O_2$.

By far the most damaging criticism of heart rate as a means of assessing the percentage of $\dot{V}O_2$ max is that absolute heart rate means little by itself. A given heart rate has meaning only relative to the individual's maximal heart rate (HR max), and HR max has great intraindividual variability. Few programs actually measure an individual's HR max. Some fitness leaders use the formula, HR max = 220 − age (in years), thus taking into consideration the well-known principle that HR max decreases with age. However, Astrand and Rodahl [8] point out that there is a 10-beat standard deviation at each age category. Therefore, a 30-year-old man with a heart rate of 160 beats per minute may, in the extreme, be working at 73 to 100 percent of HR max! The use of percentage of HR max recently was found to be a poor predictor of individual $\dot{V}O_2$ values [9].

Heart rate as a device in exercise prescription is flawed and requires a complementary means of assessing the percentage of $\dot{V}O_2$ max levels.

Ratings of Perceived Exertion

The rating of perceived exertion (RPE) is a scale developed by Gunnar Borg [10] in the early 1960s:

6		14	
7	Very, very light	15	Hard
8		16	
9	Very light	17	Very hard
10		18	
11	Fairly light	19	Very, very hard
12		20	
13	Somewhat hard		

It is very easy to use. The subject is asked simply to rate numerically the effort of the exercise, as described by Noble et al. [11]:

> Your goal is to rate your feelings which are caused by the work and not the work itself. These feelings should be general, that is about the body as a whole. We will not ask you to specify the feeling but to select a number which most accurately corresponds to your perception of your total body feeling. Keep in mind that there are no right or wrong numbers. Use any number you think is appropriate. (p. 105)

The most common criticism of the scale is that it appears to be too subjective. Because several Springfield College graduate students raised this objection last year, we set up a simple experiment for which we enlisted the aid of 10 healthy male college students who had never before seen the RPE scale [12]. On day 1, we asked them to use the RPE scale to rate four consecutive 5-minute workloads of increasing intensity on a bicycle ergometer. We then had them return to the laboratory for testing on 4 additional days. On each day, they duplicated one of the four workloads. The order of workload duplication was varied randomly among subjects. The results, shown in Table 8-1, demonstrate that the RPE is highly reliable.

To determine the value of RPE, we have attempted a thorough review of the literature in which RPE is associated with the percentage of $\dot{V}O_2$ max (Tables 8-2 through 8-4) [11, 13-24]. As can be seen in these tables, during treadmill running an RPE equal to 12 or 13 is equivalent to 61 to 86 percent of $\dot{V}O_2$ max; an RPE of 14 to 15 is equivalent to 86 to 95 percent of $\dot{V}O_2$ max; and an RPE of 16 to 17 is equivalent to 91 to 100 percent of $\dot{V}O_2$ max.

To explain the variability in RPEs of 12 to 13, we examined several very recent studies. Purvis and Cureton [13] first demonstrated that RPE is associated with anaerobic threshold. In the past year at Springfield College, Bellew [15] found that college-aged women had a mean RPE at an anaerobic threshold of 12.36 ± 1.7. Furthermore, this parameter was highly reliable (R = 0.93 and 0.98 for women and men, respectively). In another study,

Table 8-1

A Comparison of Ratings of Perceived Exertion (RPE) During Identical 5-Minute Workloads Progressively Assigned and Independently Assigned[a]

Workload (kg · m/min)	Mean % $\dot{V}o_2$ max	Mean RPE		t-Test
		Progressive Workload	Independent Workload	
300	29.9 ± 6.7	7.9 ± 1.5	8.9 ± 1.7	NS
600	43.1 ± 8.4	11.7 ± 0.9	11.5 ± 1.4	NS
900	58.8 ± 14.5	12.7 ± 1.3	13.6 ± 1.4	NS
1200	75.1 ± 14.1	16.2 ± 1.5	15.7 ± 1.6	NS

Source: Vincent et al. [12].

Note: % $\dot{V}o_2$ max = percentage of maximal oxygen uptake per minute; NS = not significant.
[a]$n = 10$.

Small [25] found the mean RPE at the anaerobic threshold to be 13.27 ± 1.6 in young runners and 13.47 ± 1.5 in middle-aged runners. The finding that RPE is related to anaerobic threshold is not surprising, since blood lactate levels also are associated with RPE [26, 27]. It follows, then, that RPE could vary within a range of levels of percentage of $\dot{V}o_2$ max, since the anaerobic threshold also varies among individuals working at the same percentage of $\dot{V}o_2$ max.

Several theories about the physiologic basis of RPE have been suggested. Two recent review articles [26, 27] are excellent. The consensus seems to call for a gestalt of factors. In some unexplained way, the central nervous system seems to process a combination of the following physiologic variables:

Lactate

pH

Carbon dioxide

Percentage of $\dot{V}o_2$ max

Heart rate

Rate of breathing

Proprioception

Temperature

Sweat

Ambient conditions

Table 8-2
Percentage of Maximal Oxygen Uptake per Minute (% V̇O₂ max) Elicited at a Rating of Perceived Exertion (RPE) of 12 to 13

Study	No., Sex, and Mean Age of Subjects	Type of Work	% $\dot{V}O_2$ max
Allen and Pandolf [14]	12 Men, 20.4 yr	Treadmill: 10 min. at 50% or 80% $\dot{V}O_2$ max	80.0
Bellew [15]	11 Men, 22.7 yr 11 Women, 21.4 yr	Treadmill: Continuous graded maximal test	M: 73.5 F: 81.0
Cafarelli and Noble [16]	10 Men, 20 yr	Treadmill: 5 min. workouts at various exercise intensities	71.0
Collins [17]	13 Men, 21.7 yr 13 Women, 20.3 yr	Treadmill: Progressive discontinuous test to exhaustion Bicycle: Identical protocol	M: 80.0 F: 86.0 M: 67.6 F: 67.5
Collins and Burke [18]	10 Women (physical education majors), 20.3 yr	Treadmill: Taylor modification; graded discontinuous maximal test	75.0
Collins et al. [19]	24 High school girls, 16 yr	Treadmill: Progressive discontinuous maximal test	86.6
Ekblom and Goldbarg [20]	19 Men, 24 yr	Treadmill: Progressive maximal test	75.0
Gamberale [21]	12 Men, 26.5 yr	Bicycle: 600 km/min	47.1
Pandolf and Noble [22]	15 Men (highly fit), 20.2 yr	Bicycle: Equivalent power outputs with pedalling speeds of 40, 60, and 80 rpm	62.0
Purvis and Cureton [13]	13 Men, 28.5 yr 17 Women, 24.5 yr	Bicycle: Continuous maximal progressive test	F: 60.3 M and F: 60.2
Sidney and Shephard [23]	26 Men, 65.2 yr 30 Women, 64.8 yr	Treadmill: 20-min. progressive walk to 90% $\dot{V}O_2$ max	M: 69.0 F: 71.0
Skinner et al. [24]	8 Men, lean, 18 yr 8 Men, obese, 18 yr	Treadmill: Progressive continuous maximal test	Lean: 61.0 Obese: 66.0
Small [25]	26 Men (experienced distance runners) Group 1: 26.1 yr Group 2: 38.7 yr	Treadmill: Progressive continuous maximal test	Group 1: 76.3 Group 2: 75.6

Table 8-3
Percentage of Maximal Oxygen Uptake per Minute (% $\dot{V}_{O_2}$ max) Elicited at a Rating of Perceived Exertion (RPE) of 14 to 15

Study	No., Sex, and Mean Age of Subjects	Type of Work		% $\dot{V}_{O_2}$ max
Burke et al. [28]	20 Highly trained swimmers 11 Girls, 14.6 yr 9 Boys, 15.1 yr	Tethered swimming: Two progressive intermittent maximal tests	F: M:	73 72
Collins and Burke [18]	10 Women (physical education majors), 20.3 yr	Treadmill: Progressive discontinuous maximal test Bicycle: Progressive discontinuous maximal test		86.4 76.7
Collins [17]	13 Men (physical education majors), 21.7 yr 13 Women (physical education majors), 20.3 yr	Treadmill: Progressive discontinuous maximal test Bicycle: Progressive discontinuous maximal test	M: F: M: F:	87.0 89.3 84.0 84.0
Collins et al. [19]	24 High school girls, 16 yr	Treadmill: Progressive discontinuous maximal test		95.1
Gamberale [21]	12 Men (healthy), 26.5 yr	Bicycle: 900 km/min		69.3
Noble et al. [11]	6 Men (highly fit), 21.3 yr	Bicycle: Three 30-min workloads at 48%, 60%, and 68% $\dot{V}_{O_2}$ max		69.5
Pandolf and Noble [22]	15 Men (highly fit), 20.2 yr	Bicycle: Equivalent power outputs with pedalling speeds of 40, 60, and 80 rpm		64.7
Purvis and Cureton [13]	13 Men, 28.5 yr 17 Women, 24.5 yr	Bicycle: Continuous maximal progressive test	M:	60.1
Skinner et al. [24]	8 Men, lean, 18 yr 8 Men, obese, 18 yr	Bicycle: Progressive continuous maximal test	Lean: Obese:	58.7 58.7

Table 8-4
Percentage of Maximal Oxygen Uptake per Minute (% $\dot{V}o_2$ max) Elicited at a Rating of Perceived Exertion (RPE) of 16 to 17

Study	No., Sex, and Mean Age of Subjects	Type of Work		% $\dot{V}o_2$ max
Burke et al. [28]	20 Highly trained swimmers 11 Girls, 14.6 yr 9 Boys, 15.1 yr	Tethered swimming: Two progressive intermittent maximal tests	F: M:	100.0 100.0
Collins and Burke [18]	10 Women (physical education majors), 20.3 yr	Treadmill: Progressive discontinuous maximal test Bicycle: Progressive discontinuous maximal test		95.1 90.1
Collins [17]	13 Men, 21.7 yr 13 Women, 20.3 yr	Treadmill: Progressive discontinuous maximal test Bicycle: Progressive discontinuous maximal test	M: F: M: F:	91.1 97.7 95.2 90.1
Collins et al. [19]	24 High school girls, 16 yr	Treadmill: Progressive discontinuous maximal test		98.5
Ekblom and Goldbarg [20]	19 Men, 24 yr	Swimming: Progressive discontinuous maximal test		100.0

When Borg [10] devised his RPE scale, the subjects he used for his study were middle-aged Swedish men working on bicycle ergometers. From the data he collected, he designed his scale such that heart rate would equal 10 times the RPE. In effect, he was using heart rate as the criterion measure for exercise intensity. Since that time, as we saw in Tables 8-2, 8-3, and 8-4, a relationship between RPE and the percentage of $\dot{V}O_2$ max has been demonstrated. Several studies have found that RPE is as good as or better than heart rate as a measure of exercise intensity [19, 28, 29].

A common criticism of RPE is that it does not work because the RPE times 10 does not equal heart rate. Recall, though, that the true criterion for exercise intensity is not heart rate but the percentage of $\dot{V}O_2$ max. Furthermore, unlike heart rate, RPE seems also to be a measure of the anaerobic threshold [13, 15, 25]. Table 8-5 describes the heart rate-RPE relationship for a sample of healthy adults in the Cornell Adult Fitness Program. As can be seen, the heart rate for RPEs of 11, 12, and 13 usually equals the RPE times 10 plus approximately 20 to 30 beats. For higher intensities, the heart rate equals the RPE times 10 plus approximately 10 beats.

Nonetheless, it is our actual clinical use of RPE which has convinced us of its effectiveness as a tool in exercise prescription. During a 4-year period in the Cornell Adult Fitness Program, following the advice of Astrand and Rodahl [8], we used principally mild interval training for the stimulus phase of the exercise periods. Following a 10- to 15-minute warm-up phase, we assigned a training stimulus of a known duration and intensity (speed). For example, on the first day, a typical training stimulus for a sedentary middle-aged man might be repetitions of a 2-minute run followed by a 1-minute walk at a pace of 75 seconds per lap (or 6 mi/hr). (For a conversion of various exercise intensities, see Michael et al. [30] p. 43.) The initial training session was based on recent exercise habits, age, sex, weight, and health

Table 8-5
Heart Rate and Rating of Perceived Exertion (RPE) During Steady-State Running in Healthy Adults

	Women[a]			Men[b]	
n	RPE	Heart Rate (beats/min)	n	RPE	Heart Rate (beats/min)
19	11	144.05 ± 12.44			
41	12	143.2 ± 18.32	41	12	160.46 ± 16.40
32	13	150.25 ± 19.36	58	13	161.83 ± 13.48
34	14	151.24 ± 19.63	31	14	167.26 ± 16.63
40	15	165.5 ± 18.83	20	15	169.30 ± 10.14
6	16	170.67 ± 20.34	11	16	174.36 ± 15.87

[a]Mean age = 32.75 ± 8.09 yr.
[b]Mean age = 29.75 ± 6.52 yr.

Table 8-6
Guidelines Found Successful in the Prescription of Exercise for Healthy Adults*

Measure of Exercise Intensity Following Exercise		Exercise Prescription
Heart Rate	RPE	
< 70% of HR max	≤ 11	*Increase* intensity, duration, or both.
70-85% of HR max	12-14	*Okay.* Increase intensity once monthly, usually in 5-second increments for each ¼ mi. Increase duration once weekly, usually one extra ¼-mi lap for each increase.
85-90% of HR max	15	*Beware.* Check heart rate. Make sure that subject is running at the assigned velocity.
> 90% of HR max	> 15	*Decrease* intensity, duration, or both. Make sure that subject is running at the new (slower) rate.

Adapted from E.J. Burke and J. Humphreys, *Fit to Exercise*. London: Pelham Books, 1982.
RPE = rating of perceived exertion; HR max = maximal heart rate.

Table 8-7
A Daily Record for the Prescription of Exercise with Sample Progression of Intensity and Duration, Each Based on the Previous Day's Heart Rate and Rating of Perceived Exertion (RPE)*

Date	Lap Time (sec) for 1/8-mi Track	Training Intervals[a]	Postexercise Heart Rate (beats/min)	Postexercise RPE
Monday, wk 1, mo 1	75[b]	2-1, 2-1, 2-1	152	13
Wednesday, wk 1, mo 1	75	2-1, 2-1, 2-1	148	12
Friday, wk 1, mo 1	75	2-1, 3-1, 2-1	148	12
Friday, wk 4, mo 1	70	2-1, 3-1, 2-1, 2-1	156	13
Friday, wk 8, mo 2	65	3-1, 4-1, 3-1, 3-1	152	14
Friday, wk 12, mo 3	60	4-1, 4-1, 4-1, 4-1	148	13

Adapted from E.J. Burke and J. Humphreys, *Fit to Exercise*. London: Pelham Books, 1982.
[a]Training intervals were divided into repetitions of 2 to 4 minutes of running followed by 1 minute of walking. The first number in each pair (e.g., 2) represents the running period and the second (e.g., 1) represents the walking period (hence, 2-1).
[b]Initial values are based on age, sex, weight, recent history of exercise, advice of physician, results of pretraining stress test, and personal interview with each participant.

status, particularly regarding the issue of cigarette smoking [31]. At the end of each stimulus period, we monitored and recorded each individual's heart rate and RPE. As shown in Table 8-6 we sought an RPE of 12 to 14 and a heart rate equal to 70 to 85 percent of the age-adjusted HR max. We wanted the exerciser to work at an RPE of 12 to 14 because this always fell within our goal of 50 to 85 percent of $\dot{V}o_2$ max (see Table 8-2). The subsequent day's exercise prescription was contingent on these goals. In this way, each day of the program was, in effect, a stress test, the results of which were used to individualize the next day's exercise program. As the sample progression in Table 8-7 shows, after 3 months of following these techniques, a healthy adult usually is running three times farther and 25 percent faster than initially at an equivalent or lower heart rate and RPE.

References

1. Clausen, J.P. Effect of physical training on cardiovascular adjustments to exercise in man. *Physiol. Rev.* 57:779–815, 1977.

2. Fox, E.L., Mathews, D.K. *The Physiological Basis of Physical Education and Athletics* (3rd ed.). New York: W.B. Saunders, 1981, pp. 293–346.

3. Saltin, B., Blomqvist, G., Mitchell, J., et al. Response to exercise after bedrest and after training. *Circulation* (Suppl. 7):1968.

4. Wasserman, K., Whipp, B., Koyal, S., Beaver, W. Anaerobic threshold and respiratory gas exchange during exercise. *J. Appl. Physiol.* 35:236–243, 1973.

5. American College of Sports Medicine Position Statement. The recommended quantity and quality of exercise for developing and maintaining fitness in healthy adults. In Burke, E. (ed.), *Exercise, Science and Fitness*. Ithaca, N.Y.: Mouvement Publications, 1980.

6. Couldry, W., Corbin, C., Wilcox, A. Carotid vs. radial pulse counts. *Physician Sportsmed.* 10(12):67–72, 1982.

7. Pollock, M.L., Broida, J., Kendrick, Z. Validity of the palpation technique of heart rate determination and its estimation of training heart rate. *Res. Q.* 43:77–81, 1972.

8. Astrand, P.O., Rodahl, K. *Textbook of Work Physiology* (2nd ed.). New York: McGraw-Hill, 1977.

9. Katch, V., Weltman, A., Sady, S., Freedson, P. Validity of the relative percent concept for equating training intensity. *Eur. J. Appl. Physiol.* 39:219–227, 1978.

10. Borg, G.V. *Physical Performance and Perceived Exertion*. Lund, Sweden: Gleerup, 1962, pp. 1–35.

11. Noble, B.J., Metz, K.R., Pandolf, K.B., Cafarelli, E.   Perceptual responses to exercise: A multiple regression study. *Med. Sci. Sports* 5:104–109, 1973.

12. Vincent, P., Makowicki, D., Burke, E.   Effects of order of exercise intensity presentation on perceived exertion and heart rate. Paper presented at the MAAHPERD Convention, Hyannis, Mass., 1982.

13. Purvis, J.W., Cureton, K.J.   Ratings of perceived exertion at the anaerobic threshold. *Ergonomics* 24:295–300, 1981.

14. Allen, P.D., Pandolf, K.P.   Perceived exertion associated with breathing hyperoxic mixtures during submaximal work. *Med. Sci. Sports* 9:122–127, 1977.

15. Bellew, K.   Reliability and Sex Differences in Rating of Perceived Exertion at Anaerobic Threshold. Master's thesis, Springfield College, Springfield, Mass., 1982.

16. Cafarelli, E., Noble, B.   The effect of inspired carbon dioxide on subjective estimates of exertion during exercise. *Ergonomics* 19:581–589, 1976.

17. Collins, M.L.   A Study of Selected Variables Related to Work Intensity. Masters thesis, Springfield College, 1982.

18. Collins, M.L., Burke, E.J.   A comparison between heart rate and perceived exertion as measures of exercise intensity in varying types of ergometry. Paper presented at the Massachusetts Association for Health, Physical Education, and Recreation Convention, Hyannis, Mass., 1982.

19. Collins, M.L., Burke, E.J., Jensen, B.E.   Comparison of heart rate and perceived exertion as measures of exercise intensity in high school females. Paper presented at the New England Chapter, American College of Sports Medicine Convention, November 1982.

20. Ekblom, B., Goldbarg, A.N.   The influence of physical training and other factors on the subjective rating of perceived exertion. *Acta Physiol. Scand.* 83:399–406, 1971.

21. Gamberale, F.   Perceived exertion, heart rate, oxygen uptake, and blood lactate in different work operations. *Ergonomics* 15:545–554, 1972.

22. Pandolf, K.B., Noble, B.J.   The effect of pedalling speed and resistance changes on perceived exertion for equivalent power outputs on the bicycle ergometer. *Med. Sci. Sports* 5:132–136, 1973.

23. Sidney, K.H., Shephard, R.J.   Perception of exertion in the elderly, effects of aging, mode of exercise and physical training. *Percept. Mot. Skills* 44:999–1010, 1977.

24. Skinner, J.S., Hutsler, R., Bergsteinova, V., Buskirk, E.R.   The validity and reliability of a rating scale of perceived exertion. *Med. Sci. Sports* 5:94–96, 1973.

25. Small, R.B.   Ratings of Perceived Exertion at Anaerobic Threshold in Young and Middle-Aged Distance Runners. Master's thesis, Springfield College, 1982.

26. Mihevic, P.M. Sensory cues for perceived exertion: a review. *Med. Sci. Sports* 13:150–163, 1981.

27. Morgan, W.P. Psychophysiology of self-awareness during vigorous physical activity. *Res. Q.* 52:385–427, 1981.

28. Burke, E.J., Meade, T. Perceived exertion during work on a tethered swimming apparatus in age-group swimmers. Paper presented at the American Alliance for Health, Physical Education, and Recreation Convention, Kansas City, May 1978.

29. Morgan, W.P., Borg, G. Perception of effort in the prescription of physical activity. In Craig, T. (ed.), *Mental Health and Emotional Aspects of Sports*. Chicago: American Medical Association, 1976, pp. 126–129.

30. Michael, E., Burke, E., Avakian, E. *Laboratory Experiences in Exercise Physiology*. Ithaca, N.Y.: Mouvement Publications, 1979, p. 43.

31. Burke, E.J., Humphreys, J.L. *Fit to Exercise*. London: Pelham Books, 1982.

IV Cardiopulmonary Considerations

9 Cardiopulmonary Exercise Testing: An Integrated Approach

Michael B. Zack, M.D.

Among the clinical reasons for using exercise testing are: measuring a patient's functional capacity, identifying coronary artery disease, developing an exercise prescription, and identifying arrhythmias. Commonly, a cardiologist will evaluate a patient by using a stress test, with careful blood pressure, electrocardiogram (ECG), and symptom evaluation, but without any measurement or collection of expired gas. Conversely, a pulmonologist will measure gas exchange, expiratory flow rates, and respiratory quotient without monitoring blood pressure and every-minute ECG strips. This parochialism of interests, although diagnostically expeditious, ignores a commonly forgotten but vitally important concept: Exercise performance always involves an integration of both the heart and the lung (as well as the circulatory, muscular, and metabolic systems). As Wasserman argues, there is no such thing as a cardiac stress test as distinct from a pulmonary stress test [1]. One always performs, in exercise testing, a *cardiopulmonary* examination.

It would seem essential, therefore, whenever we are studying exercise performance, to look at both the heart and the lung. By adding just a few measurements to the standard cardiac stress test, whether or not the exercise protocol is changed, much additional information of significant diagnostic importance can be obtained, bearing both directly and indirectly on the cardiac inquiry. Conversely, by monitoring blood pressure and the ECG during pulmonary exercise testing, patients can be spared additional exercise testing for cardiac evaluation in the future.

An ideal test is a unified comprehensive cardiopulmonary examination which would include the following measurements:

Blood Pressure Monitoring

Measuring blood pressure every minute during an exercise test identifies abnormal increases and decreases in exercise blood pressure and provides essential information about when the test should be aborted—when there is a drop in systolic blood pressure, a rise in systolic blood pressure to more than 250 mm Hg, or a rise in diastolic blood pressure to more than 120 mm Hg [2].

Electrocardiographic Monitoring

Proper 12-lead electrocardiography and three-channel monitoring during an exercise test allows detection of coronary artery disease changes, documentation of heart rate response to increased workloads, arrhythmia detection, conduction disturbance detection, and atrioventricular block recognition. It also allows the identification of the exercise test end point—when the patient is attaining 100 percent of his or her maximum heart rate, or when there is malignant ventricular ectopy or block.

Work Load Estimation

Especially when oxygen uptake ($\dot{V}_{O_2}$) is not being measured directly, it is important to identify the workload (expressed in watts) to determine at what intensity during exercise such physiologic changes as alterations in maximal oxygen uptake ($\dot{V}_{O_2}$ max), oxygen desaturation, and arrhythmias occur. It is essential that the exercise equipment (bicycle or treadmill) be properly calibrated. The workload, determined from conventional formulas or by direct measurement, at which the physiologic variables being evaluated change should be part of the data base of the examination.

Forced Expiratory Volume in One Second

Measurement of the forced expiratory volume in 1 second (FEV_1) before exercise and then again after exercise (usually 5 to 10 minutes after the completion of exercise) is a very inexpensive, high-yield procedure. A drop in FEV_1 of 10 percent or more after exercise is considered diagnostic of exercise-induced bronchospasm. This relatively common entity, which may be the sole cause of exertional limitation, can thus be easily diagnosed. It is readily treatable.

Measuring FEV_1 before exercise also allows indirect calculation of the patient's maximal ventilatory capability with exercise, his or her maximal voluntary ventilation (MVV). Multiplying the FEV_1 by 40 approximates the MVV in liters per minute. The MVV becomes the ventilatory limit to exercise performance. In normal individuals or patients with only cardiac disease, ventilation is usually not a limiting factor to exercise. In patients with lung disease, however, ventilatory limits stop exercise at levels well below cardiac functional capacity [3,4]. Patients with lung disease commonly stop at the point where their exercise minute ventilation ($\dot{V}_E$) equals their MVV.

Minute Ventilation

Measuring $\dot{V}E$ during exercise allows the diagnosis of a ventilatory limitation to exercise, when $\dot{V}E$ during exercise equals MVV and the patient stops at that point. This ventilatory limit is a ceiling above which the patient cannot possibly go. Exercising such a patient in a cardiac rehabilitation program based on conventional heart rate formulas without recognizing this ventilatory limit may create a physiologically impossible goal for the patient well in excess of his or her ventilatory capabilities, a goal that may be very dangerous, especially if the patient is also hypoxemic at this level.

Oxygenation

Traditionally, measurement of gas exchange has been accomplished by indwelling arterial catheters, sampled at various points during exercise. Of the three components of an arterial blood gas evaluation—carbon dioxide level, pH, and oxygenation—the last is the most important to measure directly. Other than for calculation of dead space measurements, arterial carbon dioxide measurements are not particularly important in exercise. Changes in pH can be inferred indirectly by identifying the anaerobic threshold in exercise (see p. 112). Oxygenation can be noninvasively assayed either by transcutaneous electrodes or by ear oximetry.

Ear oximetry can accurately determine whether oxygen (O_2) desaturation occurs with exercise. Oxygen desaturation may explain why a patient is experiencing exertional dyspnea. The ability to recognize O_2 desaturation as it occurs during exercise also provides a very important safety monitor in the test. The examiner may want to abort the test when significant desaturation occurs, as this can precede major ventricular ectopy. Just as O_2 desaturation has been shown to correlate with ECG abnormalities during sleep, so too ST-segment changes and arrhythmias on ECG can occur with exercise-induced hypoxemia. If the etiology of such ECG changes can be properly diagnosed, inappropriate therapies (such as antiarrhythmics) can be avoided and the appropriate therapy (improving oxygenation) can be instituted.

Cardiac rehabilitation patients should be prescreened to ensure that it is safe for them, in terms of adequate oxygenation, to exercise in cardiac rehabilitation units (where supplementary O_2 traditionally is not used).

Oxygen desaturation must actually be measured with exercise, since one cannot predict from resting pulmonary function tests or from arterial blood gases who will and who will not develop exercise-induced hypoxemia.

Oxygen Uptake

If the treadmill or bicycle ergometer is precisely calibrated, if the subject's efficiency in performance (stride length and frequency, walk versus jog, proper biking position and revolutions per minute, and so on) are optimal, and if factors modulating $\dot{V}o_2$ (e.g. tightness of hand grip) are minimized, then a reasonably accurate estimation of $\dot{V}o_2$ from workload can be made [3,5]. The degree to which these factors diverge from ideal represents the degree of inaccuracy of estimated rather than measured $\dot{V}o_2$. Such inaccuracy can then be replicated in exercise prescription, which commonly is based on performance $\dot{V}o_2$ or derivatives thereof, such as metabolic equivalents (METS). The collection of expired gas during exercise allows $\dot{V}o_2$ to be measured directly and correctly.

Anaerobic Threshold

The anaerobic threshold is a point in exercise when there is a greater demand for O_2 than there is supply. The anaerobic threshold probably will emerge as a reasonable parameter on which to base exercise prescription. If, in a rehabilitation context, exercise is prescribed too far below the anaerobic threshold, the patient probably will not derive the fitness adaptation sought through training. If, however, the target cardiac frequency (Fc) is set too far above the anaerobic threshold, the patient might drop out of the rehabilitation program (or worse), since the experience will be too unpleasant for him or her.

Therefore, it is useful to measure the anaerobic threshold during the exercise test and then key the exercise prescription to it, perhaps ideally setting the target Fc slightly below the anaerobic threshold Fc. Measurement of the anaerobic threshold can be obtained noninvasively by examining the slope of the curve of $\dot{V}_E$ plotted against work. If $\dot{V}o_2$ and $\dot{V}co_2$ are being measured, an even closer estimate of this point can be made.

Oxygen Pulse

Collection of expired gas allows additional cardiac information to be acquired since, strictly speaking, $\dot{V}o_2$ is a cardiac measurement. According to the Fick equation, $\dot{V}o_2$ is equal to the product of cardiac output ($\dot{Q}t$) and the arteriovenous oxygen content difference ($Cao_2 - C\bar{v}o_2$ or $C[a\text{-}\bar{v}]o_2$). Cardiac patients typically develop an anaerobic threshold at a low work rate owing to reduced stroke volume (SV), which in turn leads to reduced O_2 delivery. Other ways to identify cardiac limitation from expired gas collection are based on the Fick equation. Failure of $\dot{V}o_2$ to increase appropriately with increasing workload can occur in cardiac-limited patients if the cardiac output fails to increase.

If we substitute the product of stroke volume and cardiac frequency for cardiac output and then divide both sides of the Fick equation by cardiac frequency we arrive at the following:

$$\frac{\dot{V}O_2}{Fc} = SV \times C(a\text{-}\bar{v})O_2$$

Given the relative constancy of $C(a\text{-}\bar{v})O_2$, the term $\dot{V}O_2/Fc$, called the *oxygen pulse*, is an indirect measurement of stroke volume. Thus, the maximal achieved O_2 pulse can be compared to the predicted maximal O_2 pulse (predicted $\dot{V}O_2$ max/predicted Fc max) to assess the stroke volume competency during exercise.

Normal Values

A patient who stops exercising at a low Fc and a low $\dot{V}E$ (below MVV) without being anaerobic and without O_2 desaturation has demonstrated no physiologic limitation to exercise and could be considered to be malingering, psychogenically dyspneic, or poorly motivated. Knowledge of such information can be important clinically, particularly for disability evaluation.

Disability Evaluation

It is generally accepted that a person's job should not require more than 40 percent of his or her $\dot{V}O_2$ max. To evaluate whether an individual is subject to disability in a particular job, the subject's expired gas can be collected and $\dot{V}O_2$ max or a symptom-limited $\dot{V}O_2$ can be measured and then compared to tables in the literature [6], in which, for nearly every job, the energy cost in kilocalories or $\dot{V}O_2$ are listed. If a job requires more than 40 percent of the individual's $\dot{V}O_2$ max, either the job is too hard for that individual or the impairment that reduces his or her $\dot{V}O_2$ max can reasonably be considered to be disabling for that person and that job.

Other Diagnostic Uses of Expired Gas
Collection and Measurement

There are many other diagnostic uses of expired gas collection and measurement in exercise, including:

1. Assessing alterations in $\dot{V}O_2$-work relationships in obesity

2. Evaluating abnormalities in dead space and tidal volume with exercise in pulmonary vascular disease
3. Defining deconditioning or elite athletic achievement in terms of $\dot{V}_{O_2}$ max and the anaerobic threshold
4. Corroborating peripheral circulatory factors as limiting to exercise by a low anaerobic threshold and $\dot{V}_{O_2}$ max
5. Calculating exactly how many calories (from $\dot{V}_{O_2}$ data) are being consumed per minute at a given level of exercise and prescribing exercise based on a desired number of calories to be consumed per exercise session
6. Evaluating the efficacy of a training (normal) or rehabilitation (patient) program on the basis of improved physiologic parameters after training (decreased Fc, increased anaerobic threshold, increased $\dot{V}_{O_2}$ max, decreased $\dot{V}_E$ per workload, and so on)

Clearly, looking at the heart, the lung, and the exercising muscles together in exercise is essential in interpreting performance in normal subjects and in patients.

References

1. Wasserman, K., Whipp, B.J. Exercise physiology in health and disease. *Am. Rev. Respir. Dis.* 112:219–249, 1975.

2. American College of Sports Medicine. *ACSM Guidelines for Graded Exercise Testing and Exercise Prescription.* Philadelphia: Lea and Febiger, 1980.

3. Miller, H.S., Jones, N.L., Whipp, B.J. Guidelines for Exercise Testing and Exercise Prescription for Patients with Pulmonary Disease. Madison, Wis.: American College of Sports Medicine, 1981.

4. Jones, N.L., Campbell, E.J.M. *Clinical Exercise Testing.* Philadelphia: W.B. Saunders, 1980.

5. Astrand, P.O. Quantification of exercise capability and evaluation of physical capacity in man. *Prog. Cardiovasc. Dis.* 19:51–67, 1976.

6. Durnin, J.V.G.A., Passmore, R. *Energy, Work, and Leisure.* London: Hueneman Educational Books, 1967.

10 Basic Ventilatory Responses to Different Exercise Modalities

Timothy R. McConnell, Ph.D.
David D. Swett, Jr., M.D.
José C. Missri, M.D.
Robert M. Jeresaty, M.D.
Arfan J. Al-Hani, M.D.

There are four basic types of exercise that are used for exercise testing and training: treadmill (T), bicycle ergometry (B), arm ergometry (A), and supine bicycle ergometry (S). The latter is being used more extensively for exercise testing in conjunction with radionuclide cineangiography.

The ventilatory responses to different exercise modalities have been investigated and discussed previously [1–5]. These studies differ with respect to the equipment and protocols used. The purpose of this study was to evaluate the differences in the basic ventilatory responses to different types of exercise using protocols that are commonly employed in exercise laboratories. The implications for writing exercise prescriptions based on these results are discussed also.

Methods

Twenty healthy subjects (10 men, 10 women) between the ages of 23 and 38 years participated. Appropriate informed consent and medical clearance was obtained. Each participant performed a total of four maximal graded exercise tests using a different type of exercise (T, B, A, or S) for each test. Tests were scheduled at 1-week intervals to ensure adequate recovery between tests. The testing sequence for each subject was assigned randomly to help eliminate possible bias due to testing order.

All T tests were performed on the Quinton 1854 Cardioexercise Treadmill (Quinton Instruments Co., Seattle, Washington) using a standard Bruce protocol [6]. A Monarch 868 Bicycle Ergometer (Monark-Crescent AB, Varberg, Sweden) was used for the B tests. A similar ergometer was mounted on a table for the S and A tests. The bicycle was mounted so that the pedal sprocket was at approximately shoulder height during A. During S, the subject's feet were strapped in the pedals with the sprocket being 30 cm above table height. Protocols for B and S called for continuous 3-minute work stages with initial work rates and increments of 25 watts for women

115

and 50 watts for men. For A, an intermittent protocol was used with 2-minute work stages and 1-minute rest periods. Initial work rates and increments were 25 watts and 50 watts for women and men, respectively. All subjects were verbally motivated to continue as long as possible, and tests were terminated at the point of volitional fatigue.

During each test, the participants wore a nose clip and Hans-Rudolph breathing valve (Hans-Rudolph, Inc., Kansas City, Missouri) (100 cc dead space) held in place by a headgear apparatus. Expired air was collected and the ventilatory data was computed during each minute and at peak exercise of all tests by a Beckman Metabolic Measuring Cart (Beckman Instruments, Inc., Anaheim, California). The LB-2 and OM-11 gas analyzers were calibrated with gases of known concentrations preceding each test.

Maximal minute ventilation ($\dot{V}E$ max), tidal volume (VT max), and breathing frequency (f max) were measured at peak exercise for statistical analysis. A 2×4 factorial analysis of variance (ANOVA) with repeated measures on the second factor was computed to determine if significant differences existed between the treatment levels of the two independent variables, sex and type of exercise. Anaerobic threshold was determined for each test as the point at which the increase in $\dot{V}E$ became disproportionate with the increase in oxygen consumption or at which the ventilatory equivalent for oxygen began to increase with no concomitant increase in the ventilatory equivalent for carbon dioxide. The anaerobic threshold was expressed in absolute and relative terms. Absolute anaerobic threshold was the oxygen consumption (in liters per minute) at which the anaerobic threshold was reached. The relative anaerobic threshold was the percentage of the maximal oxygen consumption ($\dot{V}O_2$ max) at which the anaerobic threshold occurred during each test. A 2×4 factorial ANOVA was again computed to determine if any significant differences occurred between treatments for anaerobic threshold. A Newman-Keuls post hoc analysis was used to determine between which of the four types of exercise significant differences occurred. A probability level of 0.05 was used as the criterion for significance ($p < 0.05$).

Linear regression analysis was computed to determine the rate of the increase in ventilation with increasing work rate (in kilograms per minute) for men and women for each modality. The rate of the increase in breathing frequency with increasing ventilation and the ventilatory response to increasing heart rate was also computed.

Results

Table 10–1 shows the ventilatory response at peak exercise for men and women during the four exercise tests. The $\dot{V}E$ max was significantly greater during T (104.2 L/min) and B (101.1 L/min) than during S (74.3 L/min)

Table 10-1
Ventilatory Response at Peak Exercise for Men[a] and Women[a] in Four Exercise Tests

Ventilatory Factor Measured	Testing Modality				
	Treadmill (T)	Bicycle Ergometry (B)	Supine Bicycle Ergometry (S)	Arm Ergometry (A)	Mean
Maximal minute ventilation (L/min)					
Men	128.4[b,c]	123.6[b,c]	93.3	82.9	107.1[d]
Women	80.0[b,c]	78.7[b,c]	55.3	61.8	68.9
All subjects	104.2[b,c]	101.1[b,c]	74.3	72.4	
Maximal tidal volume (ml)					
Men	2729.4[b,c]	2738.6[b,c]	2175.0[c]	1826.6	2367.4[d]
Women	1914.1[b,c]	1774.6[b,c]	1463.4	1330.1	1620.6
All subjects	2321.8[b,c]	2256.6[b,c]	1819.7[c]	1578.4	
Maximal breathing frequency (breaths/min)					
Men	47.4	45.4	43.1	48.2	46.0
Women	42.0	44.1	38.3	48.6	43.3
All subjects	44.7[b]	44.7[b]	40.7	48.4[b,c]	
Absolute anaerobic threshold (L/min)					
Men	2.24[b,c,e]	1.83[b,c]	1.55[c]	1.18	1.70[d]
Women	1.25[c]	1.01	1.01	0.79	1.02
All subjects	1.75[b,c,e]	1.42[c]	1.2[c]	0.98	
Relative anaerobic threshold (% $\dot{V}o_2$ max)					
Men	56.3	51.5	53.1	43.5	51.1
Women	55.1	50.0	52.4	46.7	51.1
All subjects	55.7[c]	50.5[c]	52.8[c]	45.1	

$\dot{V}o_2$ max = maximal oxygen consumption.
[a]$n = 10$.
[b]Significantly greater than supine values at $p < 0.05$ level.
[c]Significantly greater than arm values at $p < 0.05$ level.
[d]Significantly greater than values for women at $p < 0.05$ level.
[e]Significantly greater than bicycle values at $p < 0.05$ level.

and A (72.4 L/min) for both men and women. Mean $\dot{V}$E max was significantly greater for men (107.1 L/min) than for women (68.9 L/min). The VT max also was significantly greater during T (2321.8 ml) and B (2256.6 ml) than during S (1819.7 ml) and A (1578.4 ml), and the S values (2175 ml) were significantly greater than A (1826.6 ml) for men. Mean VT max was significantly greater for men (2367.4 ml) than for women (1620.6 ml). Breathing frequency (f max), expressed as the number of breaths per minute, was significantly greater during A (48.4) than during B (44.7) and S (40.7); T (44.7) and B values were significantly larger than S values. There were no significant differences between men (46.0) and women (43.3).

The absolute anaerobic threshold was significantly greater during T (1.75 L/min) than during the other three modalities. For men, the anaerobic threshold during B (1.83 L/min) was significantly greater than S (1.55 L/min) and A (1.18 L/min), and S values were larger than A values. For the women, the absolute anaerobic threshold was significantly greater during T (1.25 L/min) than during A (0.79 L/min), with no other differences being significant. The mean absolute anaerobic threshold for men (1.70 L/min) was significantly greater than that obtained for women (1.02 L/min). When the anaerobic threshold was expressed in relative terms (the percentage of $\dot{V}O_2$ max), the values were significantly lower during A (45.1) than during the other three modalities for both sexes. There were no significant differences in mean relative absolute threshold values for men (51.1) and women (51.1).

Linear regression analysis showed that the slope of the increase in $\dot{V}E$ with increasing work rate was greater during A than during the other three modalities for both men and women (Figs. 10–1, 10–2). $\dot{V}E$ was also greater at any given work rate during A. For women, the slope of the increase in $\dot{V}E$ during T was less than that seen during B and S (Fig. 10–2). The increase in breathing frequency with increasing $\dot{V}E$ was more rapid during A than during the other three modalities for both sexes (Figs. 10–3, 10–4). Breathing frequency also was greater at any given $\dot{V}E$ during A. When the rate of the increase in $\dot{V}E$ was plotted over increasing heart rates, there were no apparent differences between the four modalities for men or women (Figs. 10–5, 10–6).

Discussion

The purpose of this investigation was to assess the ventilatory response to different exercise modalities and protocols commonly employed in exercise testing laboratories. The significantly higher $\dot{V}E$ max found during T and B when compared to S and A has been confirmed by others [1, 2]. $\dot{V}E$ max during T was 3 percent, 29 percent, and 30 percent greater than that seen during B, S, and A, respectively. These differences basically paralleled the differences found in the $\dot{V}O_2$ max between modalities. Maximal oxygen consumption during T was 10 percent, 27 percent, and 29 percent greater than that obtained during B, S, and A, respectively. Therefore, the differences in $\dot{V}E$ max values are indicative of the amount of work performed during each test. The higher $\dot{V}E$ at similar work rates and the more rapid increase in $\dot{V}E$ with increasing work rate found during A has also been reported [2, 3, 5]. Bicycle ergometry and supine bicycle ergometry appeared to cause a more rapid ventilatory response than treadmill exercise for women.

These ventilatory differences may be attributed to the fact that at each work rate the subjects were working at a greater relative work rate during

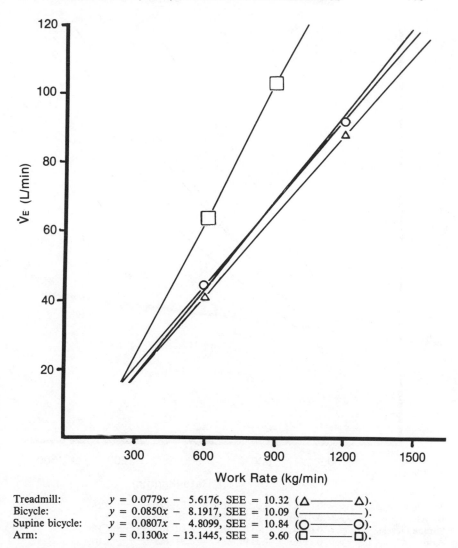

Treadmill:	$y = 0.0779x - 5.6176$, SEE $= 10.32$ ($\triangle$————$\triangle$).
Bicycle:	$y = 0.0850x - 8.1917$, SEE $= 10.09$ (————————).
Supine bicycle:	$y = 0.0807x - 4.8099$, SEE $= 10.84$ ($\bigcirc$————$\bigcirc$).
Arm:	$y = 0.1300x - 13.1445$, SEE $= 9.60$ ($\square$————$\square$).

Figure 10–1. Relationship of minute ventilation ($\dot{V}E$) to work rate for men in four types of exercise testing. SEE = standard error of the estimate.

arm exercise; therefore, a greater percentage of the energy produced would be from anaerobic glycosis, resulting in a compensatory respiratory alkalosis. That maximal breathing frequency was greater and breathing frequency increased more rapidly with increasing $\dot{V}E$ during A lends further support to this theory. At the onset of exercise, the increase in ventilation is due to a

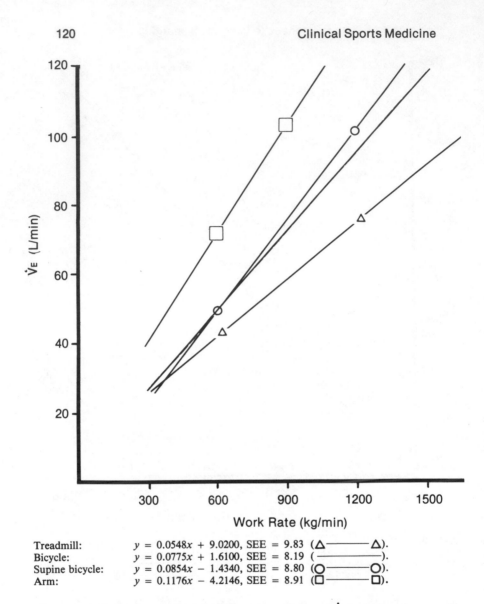

Treadmill:	$y = 0.0548x + 9.0200$, SEE = 9.83 (△————△).
Bicycle:	$y = 0.0775x + 1.6100$, SEE = 8.19 (————————).
Supine bicycle:	$y = 0.0854x - 1.4340$, SEE = 8.80 (O————O).
Arm:	$y = 0.1176x - 4.2146$, SEE = 8.91 (□————□).

Figure 10–2. Relationship of minute ventilation ($\dot{V}E$) to work rate for women in four types of exercise testing. SEE = standard error of the estimate.

more rapidly increasing tidal volume up to approximately 60 percent of $\dot{V}E$ max. Beyond this point, when metabolic acidosis develops, the continued increase in ventilation is primarily due to an increase in breathing frequency [7]. The anaerobic threshold values were obtained at a lower relative work rate during arm work, which would explain the augmented f values.

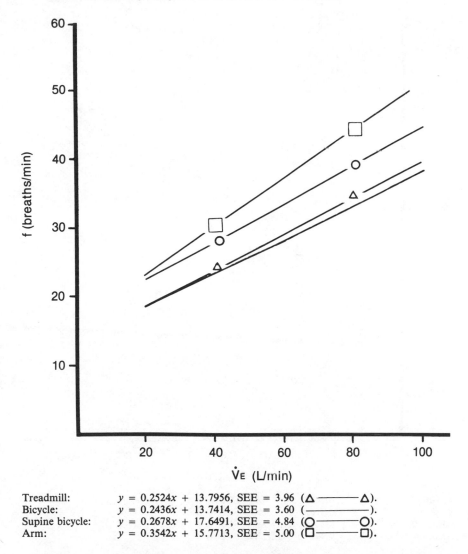

Treadmill:	$y = 0.2524x + 13.7956$, SEE = 3.96 (△————△).
Bicycle:	$y = 0.2436x + 13.7414$, SEE = 3.60 (————).
Supine bicycle:	$y = 0.2678x + 17.6491$, SEE = 4.84 (O————O).
Arm:	$y = 0.3542x + 15.7713$, SEE = 5.00 (□————□).

Figure 10-3. Relationship of breathing frequency (f) to minute ventilation ($\dot{V}E$) for men in four types of exercise testing. SEE =
standard error of the estimate.

The more rapid onset of anaerobic threshold during arm work may be
attributed to a number of factors. There may be a difference in motor unit
recruitment patterns during arm ergometry. A lack of uniform recruitment
may accelerate lactate production in the specific muscle groups involved in
the work [1]. The smaller muscle mass employed during the arm work may

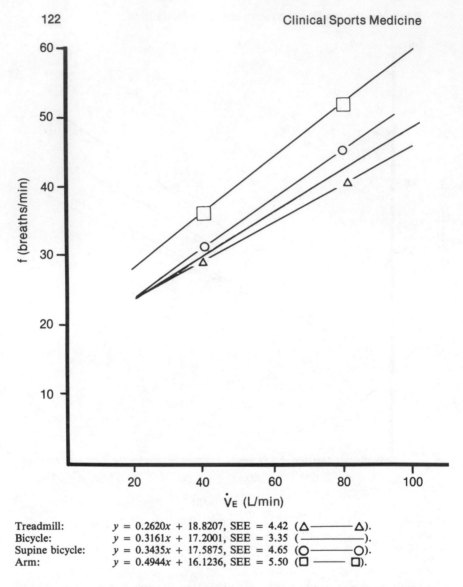

Treadmill:	$y = 0.2620x + 18.8207$, SEE $= 4.42$ (△————△).
Bicycle:	$y = 0.3161x + 17.2001$, SEE $= 3.35$ (————————).
Supine bicycle:	$y = 0.3435x + 17.5875$, SEE $= 4.65$ (O————O).
Arm:	$y = 0.4944x + 16.1236$, SEE $= 5.50$ (□ ——— □).

Figure 10-4. Relationship of breathing frequency (f) to minute ventilation ($\dot{V}E$) for women in four types of exercise testing. SEE = standard error of the estimate.

also result in an earlier onset of anaerobic threshold and fatigue. If the primary muscle groups involved in arm exercise have a greater proportion of type 2 (fast twitch) muscle fibers than the muscle groups involved during leg work, the onset of anaerobiosis would occur at a lower oxygen consumption. Differences in fiber composition between muscle groups in the

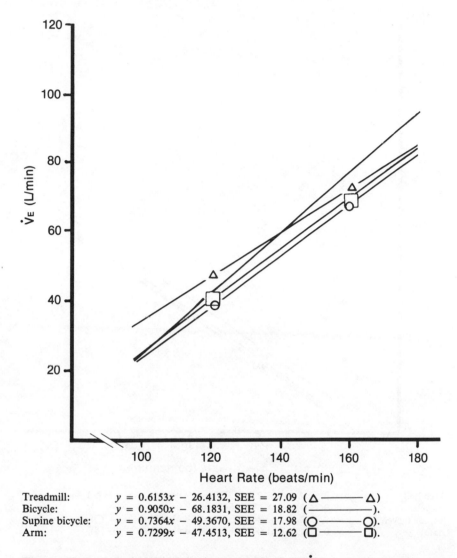

Treadmill:	$y = 0.6153x - 26.4132$, SEE $= 27.09$ ($\triangle$————$\triangle$)
Bicycle:	$y = 0.9050x - 68.1831$, SEE $= 18.82$ (————).
Supine bicycle:	$y = 0.7364x - 49.3670$, SEE $= 17.98$ ($\bigcirc$————$\bigcirc$).
Arm:	$y = 0.7299x - 47.4513$, SEE $= 12.62$ ($\square$————$\square$).

Figure 10-5. Relationship of minute ventilation ($\dot{V}E$) to heart rate for men in four types of exercise testing. SEE = standard error of the estimate.

same individual still is controversial and is under investigation [8–11]. The male participants were relatively well trained. They all ran regularly but none of them participated in regular strenuous arm work. This leg-specific training may have resulted in an enhanced oxidative capacity of the leg musculature [12–14], augmenting the differences seen between leg and arm

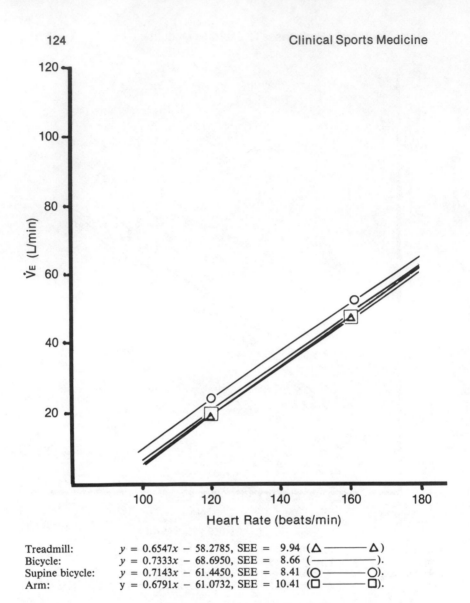

Treadmill: $y = 0.6547x - 58.2785$, SEE = 9.94 (△——————△)
Bicycle: $y = 0.7333x - 68.6950$, SEE = 8.66 (——————).
Supine bicycle: $y = 0.7143x - 61.4450$, SEE = 8.41 (○——————○).
Arm: $y = 0.6791x - 61.0732$, SEE = 10.41 (□——————□).

Figure 10-6. Relationship of minute ventilation ($\dot{V}_E$) to heart rate for women in four types of exercise testing. SEE = standard error of the estimate.

work. Also, there may have been a greater static component during arm work resulting in a decreased blood flow to the working muscle [15]. Kilbom and Persson [16] reported an enhanced pulmonary ventilation on the order of 2 to 3 L/min when a static component was added to dynamic work.

The only noticeable differences seen between men and women are that the women had a somewhat higher breathing frequency at each work rate, a lower $\dot{V}E$ at a similar heart rate, a lower $\dot{V}E$ max, and a lower absolute anaerobic threshold. These differences may all be attributed to the differences in conditioning levels between the men ($\dot{V}o_2$ max $= 57.7$ ml/kg/min) and women ($\dot{V}o_2$ max $= 40.1$ ml/kg/min). Because of this, the women were working at a higher relative work rate and had a higher heart rate response at each work increment, resulting in a lower $\dot{V}E$ at similar heart rates. The overall relative anaerobic threshold of 51.1 percent $\dot{V}o_2$ max for men and 51.1 $\dot{V}o_2$ max for women confirms those reported by others [17].

The American College of Sports Medicine's Respiratory Guidelines Subcommittee [18] recommends that a patient with a grade 2 respiratory disability train at an intensity that would elicit 75 percent of his or her $\dot{V}E$ max. At this ventilatory level during treadmill exercise, a mean heart rate of 159 beats per minute was obtained for the subjects tested. The mean $\dot{V}E$ at a heart rate of 159 beats per minute during T, B, S, and A were 58.2, 62.2, 60.6, and 56.4 L/min, respectively. These small differences indicate that the heart rate obtained at a desired $\dot{V}E$ during treadmill exercise may be appropriate for patient use in maintaining their exercise intensity at a prescribed level of $\dot{V}E$ during the other three types of exercise.

Only healthy individuals were tested. Therefore, it is difficult to discuss the clinical applicability of the data. Because the oxygen requirement for respiration increases with increasing $\dot{V}E$, it is greater at any given work rate during arm exercise. Patients with obstructive diseases have an elevated oxygen cost of breathing at any given level of ventilation [19] and, therefore, may be more limited during arm work. Breathing rates also were greater at any given level of ventilation during arm work. Because patients with restrictive diseases increase their $\dot{V}E$ primarily by increasing their breathing rates [20], they may also be more severely limited during arm work than they are with leg exercise. This is especially true since at a given ventilation an elevated breathing frequency is concomitant with lower alveolar ventilation [21].

In summary, it is apparent that the ventilatory responses to exercise differ between modalities and must be considered when selecting appropriate types of exercise for testing and training of patients with respiratory impairments.

References

1. Davies, J.A., Vodak, P., Wilmore, J.H., et al. Anaerobic threshold and maximal aerobic power for three modes of exercise. *J. Appl. Physiol.* 41:544–550, 1976.

2. Fardy, P.S., Webb, D., Hellerstein, H.K. Benefits of arm exercise in cardiac rehabilitation. *Physician Sportsmed.* 5:31–40, 1977.

3. Franklin, B.A., Scherf, J., Pamatmat, A., Rubenfire, M. Arm exercise testing and training. *Pract. Cardiol.* 8:43–53, 1982.

4. Lecerof, H. Influence of body position on exercise tolerance, heart rate, blood pressure, and respiration rate in coronary insufficiency. *Br. Heart J.* 33:78–83, 1971.

5. Smodlaka, V.N. Treadmills vs. bicycle ergometers. *Physician Sportsmed.* 10:75–80, 1982.

6. Bruce, R.A. Exercise testing of patients with coronary artery disease. *Ann. Clin. Res.* 3:323–332, 1971.

7. Levitsky, M.G. *Pulmonary Physiology.* New York: McGraw-Hill, 1982.

8. Gollnick, P.D., Armstrong, R.B., Saubert, C.W., et al. Enzyme activity and fiber composition in skeletal muscle of untrained and trained men. *J. Appl. Physiol.* 33:312–319, 1972.

9. Saltin, B., Houston, M., Nygaard, E., et al. Muscle fiber characteristics in healthy men and patients with juvenile diabetes. *Diabetes* (Suppl. 1) 1:93–99, 1979.

10. Saltin, B., Henriksson, J., Nygaard, E., Anderson, P. Fiber types and metabolic potentials of skeletal muscles in sedentary men and endurance runners. *Ann. N.Y. Acad. Sci.* 301:3–29, 1977.

11. Costill, D.L., Janies, J., Evans, W., et al. Skeletal muscle enzymes and fiber composition in male and female track athletes. *J. Appl. Physiol.* 40:149–154, 1976.

12. Herbison, G.J., Jaweed, M.M., Ditunno, J.F. Muscle fiber types. *Arch. Phys. Med. Rehabil.* 63:227–230, 1982.

13. Holloszy, J.O. Biochemical adaptions to exercise: aerobic metabolism. In Wilmore, J.H. (ed.), *Exercise and Sports Science Reviews.* New York: Academic Press, 1973.

14. Kiessling, K.H., Piehl, K., Lundquist, C.G. Effect of physical training on ultrastructural features in human skeletal muscle. In Pernow, B., Saltin, B. (eds.), *Muscle Metabolism During Exercise.* New York: Plenum Press, 1971.

15. Asmussen, E. Similarities and dissimilarities between static and dynamic exercise. *Circ. Res.* 48:I3–I10, 1981.

16. Kilbom, A., Persson, J. Cardiovascular response to dynamic and static exercise. *Circ. Res.* 48:I93–I97, 1981.

17. Skinner, J.S., McLellan, T.H. The transition from aerobic to anaerobic metabolism. *Res. Q. Exerc. Sport* 51:234–238, 1980.

18. Miller, H.S., Jones, N.L., Whipp, B.J. Respiratory Guidelines Subcommittee. *Guidelines for Exercise Testing and Exercise Prescription for Patients with Pulmonary Disease.* Madison, Wis.: American College of Sports Medicine, 1982.

19. Dempsey, J.A., Rankin, J. Physiologic adaptions of gas transport systems to muscular work in health and disease. *Am. J. Phys. Med.* 46:582–647, 1967.

20. Wasserman, K., Whipp, B.J.   Exercise physiology in health and disease. *Am. Rev. Respir. Dis.* 112:219–249, 1975.

21. Grimby, G.   Respiration in exercise. *Med. Sci. Sports* 1:9–14, 1969.

11 Hypotension After Exercise and Relaxation

Steven F. Siconolfi, Ph.D.
Richard A. Carleton, M.D.
John P. Elder, Ph.D.
Pamela A. Bouchard, M.S.N.

Exercise and relaxation each produce transient alterations in blood pressure. Hannum and Kasch [1] and Siconolfi et al. [2] have shown that systolic, but not diastolic, blood pressure decreases below preexercise resting levels following exercise. This postexercise systolic hypotension occurs in both normotensive and hypertensive individuals. Relaxation also has been shown to have a variety of effects on blood pressure. Jacobson [3], Benson et al. [4], and Bernstein and Borkovec [5] all have shown transient lowering of systolic and diastolic blood pressure immediately following relaxation therapy. We have recently shown that the combination of exercise and relaxation have a complementary effect in hypertensive patients taking beta-blocking drugs but not in patients taking diuretics [2]. In the present study, we evaluated possible mechanisms for the observed changes in systolic blood pressure after periods of exercise, of relaxation, and of exercise and relaxation in eight men with high blood pressure.

Methods

Four men with high blood pressure who were on beta-blockers (HB subjects) and four on diuretic medication (HD subjects) alone volunteered for the study. The subjects' medication usage and their general characteristics are presented in Tables 11-1 and 11-2. Prior to all testing, subjects completed a medical history questionnaire, and all their questions about the project were answered before they signed an informed consent form.

All subjects completed the four intervention protocols of exercise, relaxation, sequential exercise and relaxation periods, and a supine rest control period. These were performed at least 4 days apart. The sequence of the interventions was randomly assigned for each subject. Before each intervention, subjects rested in the supine position for 15 minutes. All physiologic and psychological measures were obtained while subjects were supine at the following times: after 5 and 15 minutes of supine rest; during the last 5 min-

Table 11-1
Anti-Hypertensive Medications of Subjects

Subject Medication

Beta-Blockers
  1. Metoprolol tartrate 150 mg
  2. Propranolol hydrochloride 120 mg, hydrochlorothiazide 25 mg
  3. Propranolol hydrochloride 120 mg, hydrochlorothiazide 25 mg
  4. Propranolol hydrochloride 160 mg, hydralazine hydrochloride 100 mg
     Allopurinol 100 mg, hydrochlorothiazide 50 mg

Diuretics
  1. Methyldopa (Aldomet) 25 mg
  2. Hydrochlorothiazide 25 mg
  3. Methyldopa (Aldomet) 50 mg
  4. Hydrochlorothiazide 25 mg

utes of the intervention; and at ½ hour and 1 hour after intervention. Between the ½-hour and the 1-hour postintervention measurements, subjects participated in low-level activities (conversation, or walking around the laboratory) prior to resuming the supine position for 5 minutes before the measurements were made.

Blood pressures were measured with a random zero sphygmomanometer (Gelman-Hawksley, Inc., London, England). This was used to reduce investigator digit bias by introducing an unknown amount of mercury into the column, which served to muddle the reading; actual readings were corrected later. Systolic blood pressure was defined as the pressure in the cuff at the time of the first Korotkoff sound. The diastolic pressure was the pressure in the cuff at the beginning of the fourth phase of Korotkoff's sounds. No results were reported to the subjects until all protocols were completed.

Heart rates were recorded electrocardiographically using a CM_5 electrode configuration. The heart rate was determined using the average of 10 beats.

Estimates of the percentage of change in total peripheral resistance (% ΔTPR) were made from the mean arterial pressure (MAP), determined as the diastolic pressure plus 33 percent of pulse pressure, and heart rate (HR), using the following formula:

$$\% \ \Delta \ TPR = \frac{[(MAP/HR)_2 - (MAP/HR)_1]}{(MAP/HR)_1} \times 100$$

This equation has been shown to produce valid and reliable estimates of changes in peripheral resistance during and after exercise [6].

Self-reported anxiety levels were recorded using the subjective units of distress scores. Subjects were asked to give a number that corresponded to

Table 11-2
Subject Charcteristics (Mean ± S.D.)

Hypertensive Subjects	Age (yr)	Weight (kg)	Systolic Blood Pressure/Diastolic Blood Pressure[a] (mm Hg)	Maximal Oxygen Consumption[b] $(ml/kg^{-1}/min^{-1})$	% Maximal Oxygen Consumption at Onset of Metabolic Acidosis
On diuretic medication (n = 4)	32 ± 7	77 ± 5	127 ± 14/82 ± 4	26 ± 2	64 ± 3
On beta-blocking medication (n = 4)	44 ± 13	89 ± 12	140 ± 10/94 ± 13	19 ± 6	67 ± 11

[a]Resting blood pressure (fourth phase diastolic).
[b]Supine exercise.

their anxiety level. They were told a 1 indicated very low anxiety (almost asleep) and 11 indicated high anxiety (for example, having just avoided a car accident). This scale, modified from a 100-point scale developed by Wolpe and Lazaurs [7], has been shown to have good internal validity.

Intervention Protocols

During a maximal exercise test, carried out between 2 and 7 days before the sequence of intervention protocols, the exercise rate for the onset of metabolic acidosis was determined using the technique described by Davis et al. [8]. The test consisted of a 4-minute warm-up period at 19.7 watts. After the warm-up was completed, the exercise rate was increased each minute by 25.5 watts until the subject could no longer continue. Measurement of minute ventilation, respiratory quotient, and the fractions of expired oxygen and expired carbon dioxide were taken during the maximal exercise test. These respiratory parameters, along with oxygen uptake, were measured with a pneumotachograph (Hewlett-Packard, Veretek Series), S-3A Oxygen Analyzer (Applied Electrochemistry, Inc.), and a Beckman LB-2 Medical Gas Analyzer (carbon dioxide analyzer). The analyzers were calibrated before each test with a gas that was chemically analyzed previously. The anaerobic threshold was taken as the exercise rate at which nonlinear increases in minute ventilation, respiratory quotient, and fraction of expired oxygen had occurred.

The exercise intervention protocol consisted of supine cycling for 30 minutes on a pedal ergometer (Warren E. Collins, Braintree, Mass.) at a work rate that approximated the anaerobic threshold onset of metabolic acidosis.

During the relaxation protocol, subjects were supine in the quiet and darkened laboratory while they used a deep muscle relaxation procedure similar to the Jacobson [3] and Bernstein and Borkovec [5] protocols. The technique is a tension-release procedure for which subjects are required to tense and then relax various muscles in their body. The sequence of tensing and relaxing was controlled by one of the investigators. The procedure lasted 30 minutes. This protocol differed from the exercise protocol in that the tension phase (lasting approximately 10 of 30 minutes) of deep muscle relaxation was a sequence of brief (6-second) short isometric contractions, whereas the exercise protocol was 30 continuous minutes of dynamic exercise.

The intervention combining exercise and relaxation consisted of 30 minutes of exercise at the rate approximating the onset of metabolic acidosis. This was followed by 30 minutes of relaxation using the procedure described previously. The intervention blood pressure with this combination was taken during the last 5 minutes of the relaxation phase.

The rest control period consisted of reading entertaining material for 30 minutes while in the supine position.

All data were analyzed as changes from the level obtained from the 5-minute preintervention rest value. Analysis of variance (ANOVA) was computed for each group. The resting values represent the difference between the values at 5 and 15 minutes of rest.

Results

The changes in systolic blood pressure, diastolic blood pressure, heart rate, percentage of change in TPR, and subjective units of distress for subjects on beta-blocking medication are shown in Table 11-3. The values for subjects on diuretic medication are shown in Table 11-4. All values are expressed as the mean plus or minus the standard error of the mean. The diastolic blood pressure showed no significant changes over time or across protocols for any group (see Tables 11-3, 11-4).

The systolic blood pressure during exercise rose significantly ($p < 0.01$) in both groups. In the HB subjects, there was a significant ($p < 0.05$) decrease (-12 ± 6 mm Hg) in systolic blood pressure below rest values ½ hour and 1 hour (-10 ± 7 mm Hg) after exercise. The subjects on diuretic medication failed to show a significant decrease after exercise. The significant increases in systolic blood pressure during exercise for both groups were associated with significant increases in heart rate ($+35 \pm 11$ beats per minute for HB subjects; $+53 \pm 4$ beats per minute for HD subjects) and significant decreases in the percentage of change in TPR ($-26 \pm 4\%$, HB; $-32 \pm 7\%$, HD). No significant changes in anxiety (subjective units of distress) were observed during exercise for either group. The decreases in systolic blood pressure ½ hour and 1 hour after exercise in the HB group were associated with decreases in the percentage of change in TPR ($-10 \pm 4\%$ and $-9 \pm 3\%$, respectively). The significant ($p < 0.05$) decrease in the percentage of change in TPR in the HD subjects during the exercise protocol also was observed ½ hour after exercise ($-13 \pm 5\%$). No other parameters were found to be significantly different from resting values for either group during or following exercise.

The relaxation protocol produced a significant ($p < 0.05$) drop in systolic blood pressure (-3 ± 1 mm Hg) in the HB subjects. This decrease was not associated with any significant changes in heart rate (-2 ± 2 beats per minute), percentage of change in TPR ($-2 \pm 4\%$), or subjective units of distress (-1 ± 1). One-half hour after the relaxation protocol, both groups showed no significant changes in systolic blood pressure, heart rate, and percentage of change in TPR. One hour after the relaxation protocol, systolic blood pressure was decreased significantly (-10 ± 8 mm Hg) for HB subjects.

Table 11-3

Physiologic and Psychological Responses to the Four Interventions in Subjects Taking Beta-Blockers (mean ± S.E.)

Intervention	Systolic Blood Pressure (mm Hg)	Diastolic Blood Pressure (mm Hg)	Heart Rate (beats/min)	% Change in Total Peripheral Resistance	Subjective Units of Distress
Exercise					
Rest	1 ± 1	1 ± 2	-2 ± 2	4 ± 2	0 ± 1
Intervention	28 ± 12[a,b]	1 ± 2	35 ± 11[a,b]	-26 ± 4[a,b]	2 ± 1[a,b]
½ hr postintervention	-12 ± 6[a,b]	-4 ± 5	4 ± 1	-10 ± 4[a,b]	0 ± 1
1 hr postintervention	-10 ± 7[a,b]	-6 ± 4	2 ± 4	-9 ± 3[a,b]	-1 ± 1
Relaxation					
Rest	0 ± 1	-3 ± 4	-3 ± 2	1 ± 5	0 ± 0
Intervention	-3 ± 1[a,b]	-6 ± 4	-2 ± 2	-2 ± 4	-1 ± 1
½ hr postintervention	-1 ± 1	-4 ± 3	-5 ± 2	5 ± 3	0 ± 1
1 hr postintervention	-10 ± 8[a,b]	-5 ± 4	1 ± 3	-1 ± 7	0 ± 1
Combination of exercise and relaxation					
Rest	0 ± 5	-2 ± 4	-3 ± 2	3 ± 3	0 ± 1
Intervention	-18 ± 4[a,b]	-6 ± 4	3 ± 4	-11 ± 7[a,b]	-3 ± 1[a,b]
½ hr postintervention	-17 ± 9[a,b]	-6 ± 5	1 ± 7	7 ± 11	-2 ± 1[a,b]
1 hr postintervention	4 ± 10	2 ± 2	-1 ± 5	5 ± 4	-2 ± 1[a,b]
Rest control period reading					
Rest	-1 ± 7	1 ± 2	-2 ± 1	-2 ± 3	0 ± 1
Intervention	3 ± 5	-5 ± 4	-2 ± 1	1 ± 2	0 ± 1
½ hr postintervention	-5 ± 4	-1 ± 3	-3 ± 1	3 ± 3	-1 ± 1
1 hr postintervention	5 ± 2	5 ± 3	-6 ± 1	14 ± 3[a]	-1 ± 1

[a] Significantly different from protocol-specific rest ($p < 0.05$).
[b] Significantly different from matched reading protocol ($p < 0.05$).

Table 11-4
Physiologic and Psychological Responses to the Four Interventions in Subjects Taking Diuretics (mean ± S.E.)

Intervention	Systolic Blood Pressure (mm Hg)	Diastolic Blood Pressure (mm Hg)	Heart Rate (beats/min)	% Change in Total Peripheral Resistance	Subjective Units of Distress
Exercise					
Rest	-1 ± 5	-5 ± 5	-2 ± 8	0 ± 7	-1 ± 1
Intervention	48 ± 9[a,b]	3 ± 6	53 ± 4[a,b]	-32 ± 7[a,b]	0 ± 2
½ hr postintervention	-6 ± 3	-6 ± 3	5 ± 6	-13 ± 5[a,b]	-1 ± 1
1 hr postintervention	6 ± 8	-2 ± 3	-1 ± 5	3 ± 6	-1 ± 2
Relaxation					
Rest	0 ± 7	4 ± 2	-3 ± 2	10 ± 6	-1 ± 1
Intervention	-8 ± 7	2 ± 2	-6 ± 3	9 ± 7	-3 ± 1[a]
½ hr postintervention	-5 ± 7	-5 ± 3	-2 ± 4	-2 ± 6	-2 ± 1[a]
1 hr post intervention	-3 ± 6	1 ± 5	-6 ± 4	-10 ± 8	-1 ± 1[a]
Combination of exercise and relaxation					
Rest	-2 ± 4	-4 ± 5	0 ± 1	-3 ± 4	0 ± 1
Intervention	-5 ± 5	-1 ± 2	5 ± 2	-10 ± 2	-4 ± 1[a,b]
½ hr postintervention	-3 ± 9	0 ± 3	2 ± 2	-2 ± 5	-2 ± 1[a]
1 hr postintervention	-7 ± 4	1 ± 3	0 ± 2	-2 ± 3	-2 ± 1[a]
Rest control period reading					
Rest	-5 ± 4	-4 ± 5	-2 ± 1	-1 ± 4	0 ± 1
Intervention	-6 ± 5	-2 ± 7	-1 ± 1	-1 ± 6	-1 ± 1
½ hr postintervention	-5 ± 8	-4 ± 6	-4 ± 2	2 ± 6	-1 ± 1
1 hr postintervention	-6 ± 6	-2 ± 7	-6 ± 2	7 ± 4	-1 ± 1

[a]Significantly different from protocol-specific rest ($p < 0.05$).
[b]Significantly different from matched reading protocol ($p < 0.05$).

No other parameters measured were changed significantly at this time for HB subjects. Subjects on diuretic medication showed no significant change in systolic blood pressure, heart rate, and percentage of change in TPR 1 hour after the relaxation protocol. However, subjective units of distress were significantly decreased for these subjects during and after this protocol.

The combination protocol (exercise and relaxation) produced a significant decrease in systolic blood pressure (-18 ± 4 mm Hg) for subjects on beta-blocking medication. This decrease was associated with a significant decrease in the percentage of change in TPR ($-11 \pm 7\%$) and in subjective units of distress (-3 ± 1). During the same intervention for the HD subjects, no significant changes were observed in systolic blood pressure, heart rate, and the percentage of change in TPR. However, anxiety levels in the HD men were significantly ($p < 0.05$) decreased during and after the combination protocol. Only a significant ($p < 0.05$) increase in the percentage of change in TPR in the HB men was noted 1 hour after the reading control period.

Discussion

The purpose of this investigation was to identify possible mechanisms for the observed changes in systolic blood pressure after exercise, relaxation, and a combination of exercise and relaxation in hypertensive men. A reading protocol was included to measure the effects of inactivity in the laboratory environment on the blood pressure response. The observed changes in diastolic blood pressure were insignificant for all protocols across the groups. This is in contrast to the findings of Shapiro et al. [9] for the relaxation procedures. The lack of significant changes in diastolic blood pressure with this protocol may reflect the sample size ($n = 8$) or may be because the relaxation procedures were done in a laboratory setting. The subjects on diuretic medication failed to show significant decreases in systolic blood pressure after any of the interventions. This may be due to the interference of the medication on the blood and to extracellular volume shifts that normally occur during and after exercise [10, 11].

Subjects on beta-blocking medication showed significant decreases in systolic blood pressure after exercise. This response is similar to that reported previously by Hannum and Kasch [1] and by Siconolfi et al. [2]. The decrease in systolic blood pressure after exercise in these groups of subjects was associated with a prolonged decrease in estimated TPR. A similar response was shown in normotensive subjects.

During the relaxation protocol, the subjects on beta-blocking medication showed a significant decrease in systolic blood pressure not shown by the men on diuretics. Although changes in heart rate, TPR, and anxiety did not reach a level of significance, all were below resting values. We postulate that the decrease in systolic blood pressure during the relaxation protocol was due to the additive effects of a decreased heart rate, reflecting a decrease in cardiac output and TPR, all related to lessened anxiety.

During the intervention and ½ hour after the intervention, the combination protocol for the HB subjects showed significantly larger decreases in systolic blood pressure than either intervention alone. During the combination, the decrease in systolic blood pressure was associated with a decrease in TPR and a decrease in anxiety (subjective units of distress). The decrease in systolic blood pressure probably reflects both a decrease in TPR (due to postexercise vasodilatation) and a decrease in cardiac output and resistance associated with lessened anxiety (the relaxation component).

Despite the small number of subjects, we suggest that both exercise and relaxation produce short-term reductions of blood pressure and that the combination of exercise and relaxation have a complementary beneficial effect in hypertensive patients taking beta-blocking drugs. Reduction in blood pressure after exercise appears to be associated with a prolonged decrease in TPR, and decreases in heart rate, cardiac output, and anxiety all contribute to the change. The decrease in blood pressure observed following the combination of exercise and relaxation appears to maximize the effects of decreased TPR from exercise and decreased anxiety from the relaxation procedure. This study suggests that patients on beta-blocking medication may obtain greater benefit from the addition of biobehavioral therapies for the control of high blood pressure than will patients on diuretic therapy.

References

1. Hannum, S.M., Kasch, F.W.   Acute post-exercise blood pressure response of hypertensive and normotensive men. *Scand. J. Sports Sci.* 3(1):11–15, 1981.

2. Siconolfi, S.F., Carleton, R.A., Elder, J.P.   Acute effects of exercise and relaxation on blood pressure (abstract). *Med. Sci. Sports Exer.* 14:181, 1982.

3. Jacobson, E.   Variation of blood pressure with skeletal muscle tension and relaxation. *Ann. Intern. Med.* 12:1194–1212, 1939.

4. Benson, J., Rosner, B.A., Marzetta, B.R., Klemchuk, H.M.   Decreased blood pressure in pharmacologically treated hypertensive patients who regularly elicited the relaxation response. *Lancet* 1:289–291, 1974.

5. Bernstein, D., Borkovec, T. *Progressive Relaxation Training.* Champaign, Ill.: Research Press, 1973.

6. Siconolfi, S.F.   Estimation of percent change in total peripheral resistance during exercise and recovery. *Cardiac Rehabil.* 2:291–296, 1982.

7. Wolpe, J., Lazaurs, A.M. *Behavior Therapy Techniques.* New York: Pergamon Press, 1966.

8. Davis, J.A., Vodak, P., Wilmore, J.H., et al. Anaerobic threshold and maximal aerobic power for three modes of exercise. *J. Appl. Physiol.* 41:544–550, 1976.

9. Shapiro, A.P., Schwartz, G.E., Ferguson, D.C.E., et al. Behavioral methods in the treatment of hypertension: a review of their clinical status. *Ann. Intern. Med.* 86:626–636, 1977.

10. Greenleaf, J.E., Convertino, V.A., Mangsett, G.R. Plasma volume during stress in man: osmolality and red cell volume. *J. Appl. Physiol.* 47:1031–1038, 1979.

11. Van Beaumont, W., Underkofler, S., Van Beaumont, S. Erythrocyte volume, plasma volume and acid-base changes in exercise and heart dehydration. *J. Appl. Physiol.* 50:1255–1262, 1981.

12 Rehabilitation of the Pulmonary Patient

Cynthia C. Zadai, M.S., R.P.T.
Colleen M. Kigin, M.S., R.P.T.

In 1942, the American Thoracic Society Council on Rehabilitation defined *rehabilitation* as "restoration of the individual to the fullest medical, emotional, social, and vocational potential of which he/she is capable" [1] (p. 663). In 1974, the American College of Chest Physicians Committee on Pulmonary Rehabilitation further qualified that concept and adopted the following as a specific definition of *rehabilitation* as it relates to individuals with respiratory disability: "Pulmonary rehabilitation may be defined as an art of medical practice wherein an individually tailored, multidisciplinary program is formulated which, through accurate diagnosis, therapy, emotional support and education, stabilizes or reverses both the physiopathology and psychopathology of pulmonary diseases and attempts to return the patient to the highest functional capacity allowed by his pulmonary handicap and overall life situation" [1] (p. 663). In this chapter, we will discuss the major facets necessary in a pulmonary rehabilitation program based on this comprehensive definition and present the current clinical applications of the most recent study findings for each.

The components of a pulmonary rehabilitation program are: selection of appropriate patients; accurate assessment of these patients, including thorough examination and diagnosis; formulation of an individual and specific course of therapy; emotional and social support; and education regarding the patients' disease and their program. The concept of pulmonary rehabilitation is not a new one, but for many years the prospects of improving or curing chronic pulmonary-diseased patients have been rather dismal. These patients seem to be a hopeless, depressed group of individuals leading sedentary lives due to extreme shortness of breath and recurrent infections. Within the last few years, because of the increased focus of medicine on exercise therapy and maximizing functional performance, these patients, despite their seemingly overwhelming disability, have been participating in and benefiting from comprehensive programs [2]. Many pulmonary physiologic parameters, specifically pulmonary function test values and arterial blood gases, still have not improved with rehabilitation, but other parameters, such as exercise endurance and the number of days spent in a hospital, are showing improvement [3].

Selecting Patients

One factor that contributes to patient success in a pulmonary rehabilitation program is the selection of an appropriate patient population. The University of Nebraska Medical Center has organized, run, and collected data from their Pulmonary Rehabilitation Program for several years. They were able to recognize some statistical trends in their successful patients versus their failures. They collected data on both physiologic and psychological parameters. Their findings show that physical indicators are more reliable than psychosocial indicators when predicting success [4]. Those patients with a forced expiratory volume in the first second of greater than 50 percent and a maximal voluntary ventilation of greater than 40 percent are more likely to improve and have success with the program than are patients with lower values. Highly motivated individuals, who want to return to a specific profession or whose jobs can be modified to accommodate the disease, have proved successful candidates despite pulmonary measurements lower than those predicted to be acceptable. Patients with histories that include a combination of physiologic problems—such as those with chronic bronchitis and heart failure or chronic pulmonary edema with recurrent infection; patients with recent life-style changes that result in rapid clinical deterioration; and patients with an inability to mobilize their psychosocial support systems—do not do as well. Although these findings can be used as guidelines, they do not preclude success in individuals with lower physiologic values or in those who require education to become motivated.

Pulmonary, Physical, and Psychosocial Examination

Each patient who is accepted and admitted to a pulmonary rehabilitation program will require a complete pulmonary, physical, and psychosocial workup. The thoracic physical examination, with attention to pulmonary musculature, is of particular importance. An understanding of the muscles of ventilation and their function and adaptation to pulmonary disease is a prerequisite for the accurate evaluation of patients and for successful program planning.

The Diaphragm

The diaphragm has recently been well described by Macklem [5]. He divides the diaphragm into two portions: the *costal* portion, innervated by branches from C-5, originating along the rib cage borders, and inserting into the central tendon; and the *crural* portion, seemingly innervated by branches of C–3 and C–4, originating from the vertebral bodies, and also inserting into the central tendon. The differences in the origin and innervation of each portion of the diaphragm allow us to look more particularly at their differences in action.

The shortening of the diaphragmatic fibers cause the diaphragm to descend onto the abdomen, increasing abdominal pressure and displacing the abdomen. The displacement anteriorly will be relative to the tone of the abdominal musculature or amount of *back pressure* the abdominal muscles are generating at any given time. Lateral abdominal displacement contributes to the lifting of the rib cage that occurs with the shortening of the costal diaphragmatic fibers. Contraction of the crural fibers contributes to increased abdominal pressure but has little effect on the rib cage motion as there are no costal attachments [5].

The intercostal musculature, which lies in sheets between the ribs, participates in the two functions of augmenting the rib cage movement created by the diaphragm and providing tone and stability for the changing pressures within the pulmonary system [6]. The accessory muscles— scalenes, sternocleidomastoids, and trapezius—are recruited during forced inspiration or exercise to both stabilize and lift the thorax, thereby increasing thoracic volume [6]. The abdominal muscles contribute to this system, as mentioned earlier, by providing tone during tidal breathing. Minimal contraction throughout inspiration creates enough back pressure to ensure that the diaphragm retains its shape and its most advantageous length to generate force. In addition, the abdominals can facilitate inspiration by contracting strongly just prior to inspiration, pushing the abdominal contents up into the thorax. By placing the diaphragm in this stretched position, the abdominal muscles can also contribute to forced exhalation by contracting strongly as the diaphragm relaxes back up into the chest [7]. Comparison of this optimally functioning system to that of the individual with chronic obstructive pulmonary disease (COPD) clarifies the disability with which we are working and aids in the planning of a treatment program.

Physiologic Alterations in Chronic
Obstructive Pulmonary Disease

The skeletal muscle's ability to function over a long period of time is related to both its strength and endurance. Muscle strength is defined as the maximal force a muscle can develop with supramaximal stimulation. Muscle endurance is determined by how long a muscle can continue to contract against a given load. Each muscle's ability to contract is also a function of its resting length. Any given skeletal muscle is at a mechanical disadvantage for generating its maximal strength when it is shortened or stretched beyond its resting length. These concepts have only recently been applied to the respiratory musculature. They are helpful when considering a patient with COPD [5].

On physical examination, the COPD patient will present with retraction of the supraclavicular spaces, widening of the subcostal angle, and an increased anteroposterior diameter or "barrel chest." The chest roentgenogram will have the characteristic appearance of an overinflated lung and a low, flat diaphragm. In addition to the airflow and gas exchange limitations of COPD patients, these musculoskeletal changes applied to the concepts of length-tension relationships, strength, and endurance are strongly indicative of why COPD patients fatigue so easily with activity. Those patients who have overinflated lungs are continually at a mechanical disadvantage. Maximal strength cannot be generated, because the rib cage and lungs are in a position of partial inflation and the diaphragm is shortened. The airway obstruction in COPD also increases the resistance to airflow, thereby increasing the workload of breathing or the strength required by the diaphragm to produce inspiration. Overinflated lungs also may shorten the accessory muscles. Summarily, COPD increases the work of breathing, and the accompanying musculoskeletal changes put the muscles at a mechanical disadvantage to respond to the work [8, 9].

We have seen the results of this type of situation in other muscles and systems. Skeletal muscles respond to a persistent increased load by hypertrophy. This is seen in the cardiac system as angina and cardiac failure when increased demand for oxygen is met with decreased supply. The long-term result of an increased demand on the pulmonary system now appears to be muscle fatigue and respiratory failure as well [5].

Muscle Fatigue and Respiratory Failure

Muscle fatigue is defined as the inability to continue to develop or maintain a predetermined force. Although the exact biomechanical mechanism of fatigue in the respiratory system is unknown, there is general agreement that when the rate of energy consumption exceeds the supply the muscle will fatigue. This principle was applied to the inspiratory muscles by Roussos et al. in 1979 [10], who studied the response of the diaphragm and the inspiratory muscles to various resistive loads. They were able to produce fatigue in normal individuals by setting a predetermined mouth pressure and having the subject attempt to maintain that pressure over a period of time. The subjects used their mouths and diaphragms initially to generate and maintain that force. However, with the onset of fatigue over time, the subjects developed a variant breathing pattern which indicated they reverted to the recruitment of accessory muscles to aid diaphragmatic contraction. Fatigue of inspiratory muscles also was produced in this study by decreasing the energy supply to the respiratory muscles or reducing the fraction of inspired oxygen below atmospheric levels in normal individuals [11].

The recruitment of accessory muscles, or reverting to alternate breathing patterns, was first described clinically in patients by Hoover in the 1920s [12]. *Hoover's sign* is an indrawing of the lower lateral rib cage on inspiration. In 1966, working with the rehabilitation of COPD patients, Innocenti [13] reported an "inspiratory bounce" in her more debilitated patients which had to be corrected with breathing retraining before these patients could exercise well. More recently, Ashutosh et al. [14] published a study documenting asynchronous breathing. They noted that in patients experiencing severe respiratory distress, there was evidence of the abdomen being alternately "sucked in" or "pushed out" during inspiration in a very irregular pattern. Macklem [5] discusses this movement in his article on diaphragmatic fatigue. Normal individuals demonstrated this activity of using first the diaphragm and then the intercostal muscles while attempting to breathe against a fatiguing load. This cyclic pattern of breathing was termed *respiratory alternans*.

Quadriplegic patients have long been noted to have an abnormal breathing pattern. In individuals with both paralyzed abdominals and little diaphragmatic activity, we see the breathing pattern known as *abdominal paradox* [5, 7]. During inspiration, the negative intrathoracic pressure is transmitted across the diaphragm to the abdomen, sucking the abdominal contents up toward the thorax and causing an inward movement of the abdomen on inspiration rather than an outward movement as seen in normal individuals. This is easily noted in quadriplegics who have flaccid diaphragms but may have to be palpated in the individual with a weak or failing diaphragm. These two abnormal breathing patterns—respiratory alternans and abdominal paradox—now are accepted as signs of fatigue and failure, respectively [5].

Evaluation Tools

The steps of physical examination of each patient prior to pulmonary rehabilitation should be intently focused on the degree of musculoskeletal adaptation to COPD. Observation and palpation will include noting the degree of supraclavicular retraction and the use of accessory musculature, use of the upper extremities to elevate and stabilize the thorax, degree of increase in the subcostal angle, ratio of anteroposterior to lateral diameter, activity of abdominal musculature during inspiration and expiration, and overall expansion, excursion, and thoracic mobility. The additional techniques of auscultation and percussion are useful to establish a baseline for each patient. Patency of the airways, presence of secretions or bronchospasm, and degree of ventilation for each individual will provide additional information as to the degree of complicating pulmonary conditions that need to be addressed in a comprehensive program. Evaluation tools in addition to the physical examination include the results of laboratory blood work, information extracted from the patient chart, stress testing as previously discussed in Chapter 9, and psychosocial evaluation scales such as the Minnesota Multiphasic Personality Inventory [15] and the Activity of Daily Living (ADL) scales [16].

Formulation of the Therapy Program

Pulmonary rehabilitation, as defined earlier, includes the aspects of assessment and treatment. After successful evaluation of the COPD patient, the selection of appropriate treatment techniques and the formulation of the proper components of the program become the priority.

Currently available treatment programs vary from strictly an inpatient 2-day treatment and teaching session to an 8-week inpatient and outpatient program with follow-up at 2 months, 6 months, and yearly thereafter. According to the American Thoracic Society (ATS) [1], the components of the rehabilitation program include bronchial hygiene and bronchodilators, breathing exercises, physical reconditioning, and oxygen use. The specific course of therapy is determined after patient selection, evaluation, and determination of goals, and before education and general considerations of smoking cessation, temperature, humidity, hydration, and nutrition [1]. Regardless of the amount of time devoted to each area, the current trend is to attempt to cover all apsects of care with a multidisciplinary team.

Bronchopulmonary Hygiene

The general purpose of bronchial hygiene is to clear out excess or retained secretions and to optimize airway dilation, thereby improving ventilation. The common components of bronchial hygiene include the use of bronchodilators (topical or systemic), with intermittent positive pressure breathing (IPPB) or aerosol nebulization; appropriate humidification; and the use of the chest physical therapy techniques of breathing exercises, positioning and the manual techniques of percussion, vibration, or shaking and cough facilitation.

Bronchodilators. The use of IPPB was standard therapy for the COPD patient population until well into the 1970s [17–19]. Common medical theory held that the COPD patient had decreased muscle ability and premature airway closure and therefore, the use of a positive pressure device would decrease the work of breathing and facilitate distribution of a bronchodilating agent. Numerous clinical trials have failed to document subjective or objective improvement in these patients with the use of IPPB. Therefore, its use has dropped precipitously [19, 20]. When use of a topical bronchodilator is prescribed, a hand-held nebulizer or air compressor now is used. For bronchodilator distribution, the hand-held nebulizer is as effective as IPPB, but it delivers medication while the patient takes a voluntary breath rather than using positive pressure [21].

Routine use of bronchodilators in the COPD population is controversial [22–24]. Their use is highly recommended for the patient who shows significant changes in airflow before and after bronchodilator use. However, for the patient who demonstrates a small immediate effect during pulmonary function testing, the use of a bronchodilator may provide therapeutic assistance which is not apparent at the testing time [23, 24]. Therefore, a therapeutic trial may often be attempted. When bronchodilators are being prescribed, the use of a topical aerosol sympathomimetic (inhaled agent) usually is the initial treatment of choice. This is due to the positive local effect of bronchodilation with few concomitant side effects. Appropriate use has been shown to improve ventilatory function as well as exercise tolerance in the COPD patient [7, 23]. With severe or persistent bronchoconstriction, the use of systemic drugs (oral sympathomimetics and theophylline derivatives) may be needed. The oral sympathomimetics now are specific to $beta_2$-adrenergic receptor stimulation and resultant bronchodilation, with little $beta_1$-adrenergic receptor cardiac stimulation. The goal of therapy is to maintain therapeutic blood levels of the agent on a routine basis with as few side effects as possible.

Chest Physical Therapy Techniques. Breathing exercises, positioning including postural drainage or bronchial drainage, and the manual techniques of percussion, vibration, or shaking and cough facilitation have long been the traditional components of pulmonary rehabilitation. In 1971, Haas and Luczak [17] published a report of a study in which these techniques comprised the entire rehabilitation program. They found that when comparing a population of 81 COPD patients receiving this treatment program to 50 control subjects receiving only symptomatic treatment of bronchodilators, oxygen delivery, and IPPB, the rehabilitation group had increased exercise ability in walking, climbing stairs, and weaving, as well as decreased oxygen debt and decreased recovery time during exercise testing. Other investigators also emphasize the importance of this type of treatment within the scope of the rehabilitation program [25–27]. Shapiro and Vostinak [27] felt that bronchial hygiene was a significant factor in the physiologic and subjective improvement of 40 patients who went through a 2-year rehabilitation program.

The precise use and effects of postural drainage and percussion, vibration, or shaking and cough facilitation have been further investigated and reviewed for the COPD population [23a, 28, 29]. Despite the evidence of positive effects found by some investigators, the proper use of these techniques within the context of pulmonary rehabilitation remains unclear. The presence of excess retained secretions should be documented for each patient. Patients without secretions do not seem to warrant this component of care. A careful history as well as physical examination and, in questionable situations, a trial use, will help clarify the need or potential benefit of this type of therapy. It is unknown whether the production of 30 ml of sputum or more, as espoused by Murray [30], is necessary to receive benefit from these techniques or whether retention of smaller amounts of secretion over a long period of time would deleteriously affect the rapid progression of the disease or the number of chest infections per year.

Cough is a critical element of the treatment to remove the excess retained secretions. The COPD patient often experiences difficulty achieving an effective cough, most likely due to a combination of premature airway collapse and weakened pulmonary musculature. Therefore, such patients frequently labor to remove secretions using long periods of coughing or regular clearing of the throat. Some patients have noted that "huffing" (a forced expiration technique) is an easier and effective method of clearing secretions. This technique has been studied in subjects with chronic lung disease, including those with asthma and cystic fibrosis [31, 32]. These researchers concluded that huffing is an effective means of mobilizing secretions and may provide better stabilization of the airways than does coughing. The benefit of providing instruction in coughing after exercise has been noted in our clinic. Patients must be instructed to move out loosened secretions in a controlled, energy-efficient manner.

Breathing Exercises

Breathing exercises have been used for many years in the treatment of COPD. During the 1930s, Winnifred Linton described the techniques of breathing retraining [33]. In the 1960s and early 1970s, the technique of "pursed-lip breathing" was examined as many COPD patients adopted the pattern on their own and found it beneficial for use during exercise and periods of stress [34, 35]. Various researchers also were examining the respiratory rate and pattern of breathing, including inspiratory time versus expiratory time and the effect that different rates and patterns had on gas mixing and improving oxygenation [36–38]. In addition, during that decade, clinicians and researchers noted that performance and exercise seemed dependent on a pattern of breathing, the use of the musculature, and the capabilities of the muscles themselves [39]. In 1976, Leith and Bradley [40] published a landmark study documenting that the respiratory muscles responded to exercise and could be trained for strength and endurance as are other skeletal muscles. Since that time, so-called breathing exercises have been looked on in a totally different way.

The study by Leith and Bradley [40] involved normal subjects in laboratory conditions. Four individuals trained against an inspiratory resistance, attempting greater and greater amounts of force. Four other subjects trained using the maximal voluntary ventilation maneuver, patterned breathing at a predetermined level, and performed this maneuver for measured amounts of time. The first group of volunteers significantly increased the strength of their inspiratory muscles measured by the force generated. The second group significantly increased their endurance based on the measured volume of air they moved over time. These increases in strength and endurance, however, were not transferable. Both groups retained their pretraining values in the opposing category. The questions these findings generate include: Can these methods be adapted to the clinical setting? Are these results possible in the patient population? If the answer to these questions is "yes," we then can ask, "Does this type of training have beneficial effects for the COPD patient?"

Keens et al. [41] in 1977 studied cystic fibrosis (CF) patients in the unlikely clinical setting of summer camp. The subjects were divided into two training groups and one control group. The first CF group trained in methods similar to those developed by Leith and Bradley [40], using hyperpnea to increase muscle strength and endurance. The second group of CF subjects simply participated in camp activities, including 2 or 3 hours daily of swimming, rowing, and canoeing in particular, as well as the remaining camp program. After 4 weeks, both CF groups demonstrated increased ventilatory strength and endurance.

In 1982, Asher et al. [42] did further work with CF patients. These investigators developed an alternative method of training. Rather than training for strength or endurance against an occluded airway or with hyperpnea, these patients performed "training runs" against an inspiratory resistance device. By increasing resistance to airflow and having the patient breathe for a measured amount of time, both strength and endurance were measured. The results of this study showed that, although there was a significant increase in both the strength and endurance of ventilatory muscles, there was not demonstrable improvement in mean exercise performance during either progressive or submaximal exercise testing [42]. Several other studies in the last 2 years have examined similar questions with different populations and different results (Table 12-1) [43–46]. From these findings we may conclude that inspiratory muscle training (IMT) as a form of breathing exercise can improve strength and endurance of inspiratory

Table 12-1
Results of Inspiratory Muscle Training (IMT)

Researchers	Patient Population	Method and Length of Training	Findings
Pardy et al. [43]	17 Patients, chronic airflow limitation	9 Patients: Control (variant exercise) group 8 Patients: Inspiratory muscle resistive training, 30 minutes daily	After 1 month, control group increased distance covered during 12-minute walk, but no further increase was seen in exercise performance with training. However, attendance was not regular, and duration and intensity of exercise was not standard. The IMT group increased both endurance time and distance covered during 12-minute walk.
Pardy et al. [44]	12 Patients, moderate to severe chronic airflow limitation	Inspiration against a previously determined critical resistance for two 15-minute sessions daily. Tests repeated at 1 and 2 months' training	All showed increased respiratory muscle endurance but no increase in strength. Seven of 12 patients increased endurance time for submaximal exercise. Of those, 6 had electromyographic changes indicating inspiratory muscle fatigue on pretraining submaximal exercise tests.
Belman and Mittman [45]	10 Patients with COPD	6-Week training program, with two 15-minute MSVC runs per day and 15 minutes of rest between each attempt (hyperpnea)	No significant changes in lung volumes or spirometric indexes. Significant increases in: MSVC and MSVC/FEV$_1$; oxygen consumption during MSVC; MSVC heart rate; maximal exercise ventilation for both arm and leg exercise; endurance time at a submaximal workload; and maximal distance covered with a 12-minute walk.
Belman and Kendregan [46]	15 patients with COPD	8 Patients: Arm ergometry, 6 weeks 7 Patients: Leg ergometry, 6 weeks	No significant changes in lung volumes or spirometric indexes. Significant increases in mean endurance workload for 20 minutes per arm and leg. No significant change in MSVC for arm or leg trainees.

COPD = chronic obstructive pulmonary disease; MSVC = maximal sustainable ventilatory capacity; FEV$_1$ = forced expiratory volume in the first second.

muscles with either inspiratory resistance training or the hyperpnea method. This training may or may not improve exercise performance, depending on the method used, the degree of inspiratory muscle fatigue initially, and the patient population. There remains a question as to whether exercise training can increase strength and endurance of ventilatory muscles, although with some methods and populations, the results seem to indicate that this is possible.

Once the decision to use breathing exercises has been made and the methods have been selected, there are other decisions to be made regarding their place within the rehabilitation program. Some researchers have begun to place breathing training in a comprehensive program, using all the components listed by the ATS [1], and others have attempted to replace their comprehensive programs with IMT alone. It is interesting to examine the findings of Casciari et al. [47], who compared two groups of COPD patients, one group participating in an exercise conditioning program and the second group in an exercise conditioning program with breathing retraining. (Breathing retraining is described in Table 12–1.) Both groups participated in a control period of training, and subjects were closely matched for ventilatory values. Their medical management, including the use of bronchodilators, antibiotics, diuretics, digitalis, and oxygen therapy, was also similar. Significant differences between the groups were seen only after Group 2 added the breathing retraining to their program. The changes noted were an increased resting oxygen consumption, decreased resting respiratory rate as well as decreased respiratory rate during maximal exercise, increased tidal volume during maximal exercise, and increased arterial oxygenation during exercise. This study raises questions about what types of exercise and other treatment components comprise the most successful pulmonary rehabilitation program.

Physical Reconditioning

Exercise training to promote endurance through maximizing the efficiency of the cardiopulmonary system by decreasing oxygen extraction and increasing cardiac output per stroke volume has been addressed for years in the sports arena and more recently in relation to disabilities including cardiac disease [48]. The use of exercise for patients with COPD has not been widespread until recently, and, in fact, patients often were advised to minimize all activity and to retire on disability benefits.

In 1952, Barach [49] was the first to emphasize maintained ambulation and activity of COPD patients, having noticed that the active patients appeared to function better than their inactive counterparts. Since that time, numerous studies on the effects of exercise for COPD patients have been done, using a variety of exercise modes, intensities, durations, and frequencies, and various types of patients (Table 12-2) [25, 50-57]. A wide variety of findings have been recorded, but consistently, regardless of exercise mode or patient type, an increased ability to exercise with decreased oxygen consumption has been documented [50-52]. The study findings also show an inconsistent pattern of changing ventilatory function or lung volume measured through pulmonary function tests, but generally there is no change [25, 49, 54]. Proposed reasons for the increased exercise ability without change in lung function include: decreased sensitivity to dyspnea; decreased oxygen cost of breathing through a controlled, coordinated ventilatory pattern; general increased coordination in movement; and increased peripheral oxygen use due to increased peripheral blood flow [22].

In 1981, Belman and associates [58, 59] were the first to measure the effects of training on the skeletal muscles of COPD patients through muscle biopsies of the untrained and trained extremities. They found no increase in mitochondrial enzymes, as is found in normal subjects after training. In a normal person, heart rate changes appear to be linked to peripheral muscle changes [59]. In the COPD population, studies vary as to changes in heart rate [58]. Belman [59] indicates that a lack of change in heart rate plus peripheral changes is consistent with the theory that these patients do not attain an aerobic threshold to achieve a true training response.

Training Modes. The methods of training have varied from use of a treadmill, bicycle erogometer, stair climbing, or walking to jogging, swimming, and caonoeing in the cystic fibrosis population. A particular exercise mode is selected for a variety of reasons, including availability of equipment, space, the patient's musculoskeletal status (for example, a patient with arthritis or a prior hip or knee injury would not use the treadmill or walking but could use an ergometer), ease in monitoring, and specificity of training effects.

In 1966, Paez [51] attempted to study specificity of training in COPD patients. He trained eight patients on a treadmill for 3 weeks. All patients had an increased walking capacity, decreased pulse rate, and lengthening of stride after training. With ergometry testing before and after treadmill training, he concluded that the improvement of these patients was greatest when the patients were participating in a form of exercise they were trained to do. This information matches that available for the training of normal individuals [48].

Despite the establishment of group exercise programs, patients must be evaluated for their individual training needs as well as their musculoskeletal status to determine the best mode of exercise. The COPD patient is being rehabilitated to allow for an increase in activity. If the patient's restriction is an inability to walk, then it is logical that the training mode should be the treadmill or flat-surface walking. Many programs do not have access to a treadmill for testing or training, and therefore a program is established using flat-surface walking in combination with ergometry before and after testing and training. Whichever training mode is used, attention should be paid to pretraining and posttraining evaluation of the patient's ability to participate in activities of daily living. Scales are available for such evaluation [16]. Table 12-3 is an example of such a scale. If a bicycle program alone is used, it is necessary to observe the patient's walking pattern as well. A home program of walking may also have to be included. Increased exercise ability on any type of equipment is not useful if the patient cannot also increase activities of daily living with equal ease.

Intensity, Frequency and Duration of Training. The intensity, frequency, and duration of training programs vary dramatically (see Table 12-2). The

Table 12-3
Sample Scale for Evaluating a Patient's Ability to Participate in Activities of Daily Living: Functional Status Index

Activity	Assistance $(1 \rightarrow 5)$[a]	Dyspnea $(0 \rightarrow 7)$[b]	Difficulty $(0 \rightarrow 7)$[c]	Comments
Mobility				
Walking inside	_____	_____	_____	
Climbing up stairs	_____	_____	_____	
Transferring to and from toilet	_____	_____	_____	
Getting in and out of bed	_____	_____	_____	
Driving a car	_____	_____	_____	
Personal care				
Combing hair	_____	_____	_____	
Putting on pants	_____	_____	_____	
Buttoning clothes	_____	_____	_____	
Washing all parts of the body	_____	_____	_____	
Putting on shoes or slippers	_____	_____	_____	
Home chores				
Vacuuming a rug	_____	_____	_____	
Reaching into high cupboards	_____	_____	_____	
Doing laundry	_____	_____	_____	
Washing windows	_____	_____	_____	
Doing yard work	_____	_____	_____	
Hand activities				
Writing	_____	_____	_____	
Opening containers	_____	_____	_____	
Turning faucets	_____	_____	_____	
Cutting food	_____	_____	_____	
Vocational				
Performing all job responsibilities	_____	_____	_____	
Avocational				
Performing hobbies requiring hand work	_____	_____	_____	
Attending church	_____	_____	_____	
Socializing with friends and relatives	_____	_____	_____	

Source: Scale developed by Jette [15]. © AMJ 1980.
Note: Time Frame—on the average during the past (7) days.
[a]1 = independent; 2 = uses devices; 3 = uses human assistance; 4 = uses devices and human assistance; 5 = unable to do.
[b]0 → 7, where 0 = no dyspnea and 7 = extremely severe dyspnea.
[c]0 → 7, where 0 = not difficult and 7 = extremely difficult.

Table 12-2
Results of Exercise Training in Patients with Chronic Obstructive Pulmonary Disease

Study[a]	Length of Training	Type of Training	O_2 Consumption	Heart Rate	Respiratory Rate	Pulmonary Function Tests	Maximal Workload
Miller et al. [50] (n = data not given)	6 wk	Treadmill, 2½-min maximal tolerated level once or twice daily	Decreased 25%	Decreased	Decreased 40%	No change	Not evaluated in maximal terms, but by 50% greater tolerance of treadmill speed, had 30% greater maximal O_2 uptake
Woolf and Suero [52] (n = 14)	1 mo without O_2 2 mo with O_2	Walk for 30 min at 1 mph on a four-degree grade once or twice daily	Decreased		Decreased, became deeper with training	Increased physiologic deadspace	
Bass et al. [53] (n = 11)	18 wk	Ergometry, 20 min three times daily, graded load	Decreased	Decreased at rest and during exercise		Increased maximal voluntary ventilation ($p < 0.05$); increased inspiratory capacity ($p < 0.05$)	Increased

Study	Duration	Program				
Vyas et al. [55] (n = 11)	6–26 wk	Ergometry, warm-up for 5 min at 60 kg/min; then 1–2 min exercise at 90% maximal tolerated level two times per session daily	Improved 10%			Increased
Laros and Swierenga [54] (n = data not given)	7 mo	Ergometry, 3-min periods at 40% maximal workload four times weekly; exercise to tolerance as program progressed		Decreased		
Brundin [25] (n = 31)	4–12 mo	Ergometry, at submaximal level— 4 min of work, 4 min of rest—once or twice every 2 wk		No change	No consistent change	
Smodlaka and Adamovich [56] (n = 27)	3–6 mo	Ergometry, 30 sec of work, 60 sec of rest, repeated during 45-min sessions two to three times weekly	Decreased	No change relative to work capacity		

[a] All subjects were diagnosed as having chronic obstructive pulmonary disease.

basic principles of training apply to the COPD patient as well as to the athlete: The individual should optimally be subjected to a training level of sufficient intensity, frequency, and duration to produce measurable change. The person must be subjected to overload, a stress greater than what is experienced in activities of daily living [48]. It must be remembered that for athletes, the more physically fit they are, the more it will take to improve their fitness, whereas for the COPD population, which is extremely debilitated, any increase in activity appears to produce measurable change. That the COPD population may not achieve an aerobic threshold with training must also be remembered [58].

Intensity. The intensities of various training programs have varied from submaximal to maximal, and the duration from short-term training to 1 hour of continuous activity. Examples of these diverse programs include the following:

> Thirty seconds of work followed by 60 seconds of rest, 30 repetitions per session, 45-minute sessions, three times per week on a bicycle (interval training) [56]

> Two and one-half minutes at maximal workload one to two times per day on a treadmill [60]

> Ten minutes per day at submaximal level, five times daily on a bicycle [50]

> Three 10-minute walks per session, three times per week, with walks 1 and 3 at maximal workloads and walk 2 at submaximal load [26]

> One hour of walking daily at submaximal workload, using a combination of treadmill, hall walking, and stair climbing [39]

Patients often are encouraged to walk in the halls or at home in addition to completing their training activities [51].

Frequency. In established programs, training sessions have ranged from five times per day [51] to as infrequently as once every 2 weeks [25]. In fact, a purpose of Brundin's [25] every-2-week program was to evaluate limited formal training. These patients increased their exercise tolerance, and Brundin concluded that patients can get positive results from infrequent training with long sessions and continued activity between sessions.

Duration. The length of training programs ranges from 3 to 6 weeks up to 18 months. A few conclusions have been drawn by investigators regarding the length of formal training. Nicholas et al. [26], in 1970, reported about a program that consisted of a 3-month control period (bronchial hygiene plus one time per week walking on a treadmill just to establish a walking score) and a 6-month training program (consisting of three 10-minute walks three times weekly, with walks 1 and 3 at maximal workload and walk 2 at submaximal workload). The majority of changes in patient exercise ability were recorded within the first 3 months, although one patient continued to improve in exercise tolerance throughout the 6-month span. Subjects all had a forced expiratory volume in the first second of less than 1 L/min; oxygen tension of 61 to 100 mm Hg; and carbon dioxide tension of 34 to 58 mm Hg at rest. The investigators concluded that the length of the study contributed to a high dropout rate and that the overall results indicate a short course of therapy (2 to 3 months) would accomplish the maximal increase observed in most subjects [26].

Use of Oxygen. Recognizing the possibility for oxygen desaturation that some COPD patients experience with activity, some programs employ low-flow oxygen during exercise sessions. Other programs use oxygen only for patients who show desaturation during the exercise testing. Woolf and Suero [52] exercised patients without supplemental oxygen two times per day until they were able to walk at a rate of 1 mph on a four-degree grade for 30 minutes on a treadmill. They found 8 participants (of 14) who could reach a maximum of only 4 minutes of exercising and could progress no further. To these patients, they administered 60% oxygen during exercise and trained the patients until they could walk for 30 minutes at 1 mph on a four-degree grade. Those patients who did not need supplemental oxygen for continued improvement reached the 30-minute goal in approximately 1 month, whereas those who leveled off and needed oxygen required approximately 2 months to accomplish the 30-minute walk.

Changes Expected with an Exercise Program. As mentioned previously, the changes expected in pulmonary patients on an exercise program include increased work tolerance, decreased oxygen consumption per unit workload, decreased respiratory rate, and according to some studies, a decrease in heart rate. No consistent changes in pulmonary function tests have been seen, but indications for a decline in progression have been noted [39]. With these physiologic changes, investigators have noted a decrease in the number of days a patient is hospitalized and an increase in the quality of life [27]. The low documentation regarding return to work has been attributed to the severity of illness and age of the patients who are traditionally participating in these programs. There has recently been an attempt to enter younger, less severely ill patients in these programs, and there is hope that this trend will continue.

Psychosocial Support

Chronic pulmonary patients are most often debilitated by a severe and recurrent disease process. Frequently, they react with signs of denial, depression, anger, and anxiety. These psychological reactions and behaviors can critically affect the success of a rehabilitation program. Therefore, appropriate counseling is a necessary component of the rehabilitation program [23]. These patients often have a realistic recognition of the severity of their illness, and therapy to promote insight into their disease may not provide for a change in their feelings [24]. Drug therapy to counter depression must be carefully considered, due to the potential risk of the sedating effects of such drugs [24]. Scales may be used to establish a patient's baseline feelings, allowing for documentation of change with rehabilitation, such as a decrease in depression and anxiety [2]. Psychosocial support alone, however, does not provide for the increased activity that a combination of psychosocial support and exercising promotes [18].

Nutrition

An area often overlooked yet critically important for chronic pulmonary patients is an adequate nutritional program. Sufficient food intake for daily activities is sometimes a problem. An exercise program imposes additional food requirements. A nutritional assessment and dietary program should be provided for patients who are either overly obese or undernourished due to the disease. Obesity can increase the work of breathing. Arora and Rochester [61] recently reported on the decreased respiratory muscle strength and maximal voluntary ventilation in undernourished patients with pulmonary disease when compared to well-nourished patients with pulmonary disease. They concluded that reduced respiratory muscle endurance, which increases the work of breathing, might predispose patients with COPD to premature development of respiratory failure.

Patient Education

The inclusion of patient education is considered critical to the success of any pulmonary rehabilitation program [23]. Educational elements of a program include patient and family instruction in pulmonary anatomy and physiology, the use of medications, including their action and side effects, the care of equipment, bronchial drainage techniques, and nutritional needs and support.

There is apparently no difference in the amount learned if the patient is taught individually, in a group, or through written explanation [62]. Perry [63] found a significant increase in learning in the COPD patient while employing the learning principles that develop the patient's need to learn, provide a conducive learning environment, and promote patient participation. He measured learning through use of a patient diary that included a recording of symptoms and treatment and perceptions of decision making and daily activities.

References

1. American Thoracic Society. Pulmonary rehabilitation: Official ATS statement. *Am. Rev. Respir. Dis.* 124:663, 1981.

2. Petty, T.L. Pulmonary rehabilitation. *Am. Rev. Respir. Dis.* 122:159, 1980.

3. Hudson, L.D., Tyler, M.L., Petty, T.L. Hospitalization needs during an outpatient rehabilitation program for chronic airway obstruction. *Chest* 70:607, 1976.

4. Kass, I., Dyksterhuis, J.E., Rubin, H., et al. Correlations of psychophysiological variables with vocational rehabilitation outcome in patients with chronic obstructive pulmonary disease. *Chest* 67:433, 1975.

5. Macklem, P.T. The diaphragm in health and disease. *J. Lab. Clin. Med.* 99:601, 1982.

6. Danon, J., Drug, W.S., Goldberg, N.B., Sharp, J.T. Function of the isolated paced diaphragm and the cervical accessory muscles in C1 quadriplegics. *Am. Rev. Respir. Dis.* 119:909, 1976.

7. Luce, J.M., Culver, B.H. Respiratory muscle function in health and disease. *Chest* 81(1):82, 1982.

8. Roussos, C.S., Fixby, M.S., Gross, D., Macklem, P.T. Respiratory muscle fatigue in man at FRC and higher lung volumes (abstract). *Physiologist* 19:345, 1976.

9. Sharp, J.T., Drutz, W.S., Moisan, T., et al. Postural relief of dyspnea in severe chronic obstructive pulmonary disease. *Am. Rev. Respir. Dis.* 122:201, 1980.

10. Roussos, C., Fixley, M., Gross, D., Macklem, P.T. Fatigue of inspiratory muscles and their synergistic behavior. *J. Appl. Physiol.* 46:897, 1979.

11. Roussos, C., Macklem, P.T. Diaphragmatic fatigue in man. *J. Appl. Physiol.* 43:189, 1977.

12. Hoover, C.F. Definitive percussion on and inspection in estimating the size and contour of the heart. *J.A.M.A.* 75:1625, 1920.

13. Innocenti, D. Breathing exercises in the treatment of emphysema. *Physiotherapy* 52:437, 1966.

14. Ashutosh, K., Gilbert, R., Auchincloss, J., Peppi, D. Asynchronous breathing movements in patients with chronic obstructive pulmonary disease. *Chest* 67(5):553, 1975.

15. Jette, A. The functional status index: reliability of a chronic disease evaluation instrument. *Arch. Phys. Med. Rehabil.* 61:395, 1980.

16. Moser, K.M., Bokinsky, G.E., Savage, R.T., et al. Results of a comprehensive rehabilitation program. *Arch. Intern. Med.* 140:1596, 1980.

17. Haas, A., Luczak, A. The importance of rehabilitation in the treatment of chronic pulmonary emphysema. *Arch. Phys. Med. Rehabil.* 42(11):733, 1961.

18. Lustig, F.M., Castillo, R., Haas, A.   Rehabilitation regime in patients with chronic obstructive pulmonary diseases. *Arch. Phys. Med. Rehabil.* 54:315, 1972.

19. Murray, J.F.   Review of the state of the art in intermittent positive pressure breathing therapy. *Am. Rev. Respir. Dis.* 110(Suppl.):193, 1974.

20. Hodgkin, J.E.   Chronic obstructive airway diseases: current concepts in diagnosis and comprehensive care. *J.A.M.A.* 232(12):1243, 1975.

21. Cherniack, R.M.   Intermittent positive pressure breathing in management of chronic obstructive pulmonary disease: current state of the art. *Am. Rev. Respir. Dis.* 110(6):188, 1974.

22. Carasso, B.   Therapeutic options in COPD. *Geriatrics* 37(5):99, 1982.

23. Lertzman, M.M., Cherniack, R.M.   State of the art: rehabilitation of patients with chronic obstructive pulmonary disease. *Am. Rev. Respir. Dis.* 114:145, 1976.

23a. Pham, Q.T., Peslin, R., Puchelle, E., et al.   Respiratory function and the rheological status of bronchial secretions collected by spontaneous expectoration and after physiotherapy. *Bul!. Physiopathol. Respir.* 9:293, 1973.

24. McDonald, G.L., Hudson, L.D.   Important aspects of pulmonary rehabilitation. *Geriatrics* 37(3):127, 1982.

25. Brundin, A.   Physical training in severe chronic obstructive lung disease: I. Clinical course, physical working capacity and ventilation. *Scand. J. Respir. Dis.* 15:25, 1974.

26. Nicholas, J.J., Gilbert, R., Gabe, R., Auchincloss, J.H., Jr.   Evaluation of an exercise therapy program for patients with chronic obstructive pulmonary disease. *Am. Rev. Respir. Dis.* 114:1–9, 1970.

27. Shapiro, B.A., Vostinak, E.J.   Respiratory therapy techniques in pulmonary rehabilitation (abstract). *Arch. Phys. Med. Rehabil.* 57(11):560, 1976.

28. Anthonisen, P., Rus, P., Sgaard-Andersen, T.   The value of lung physical therapy in the treatment of acute exacerbations of chronic bronchitis. *Acta Med. Scand.* 175:715, 1964.

29. Bateman, J.R.M., Newman, S.P., Daunt, K.M., et al.   Regional lung clearance of excessive bronchial secretions during chest physiotherapy in patients with stable chronic airways obstruction. *Lancet* 1:294, 1979.

30. Murray, J.F.   The ketchup bottle method (editorial). *N. Engl. J. Med.* 300(20):155, 1979.

31. Pryor, J.A., Webber, B.A.   An evaluation of the forced expiration technique as an adjunct to postural drainage. *Physiotherapy* 65(10):304, 1979.

32. Thompson, B., Thompson, H.T.   Forced expiratory exercises in asthma and their effect on FEV_1. *N. Z. J. Physiother.* 3(15):19, 1968.

33. Gaskell, D.V.   *Physiotherapy for Medical and Surgical Thoracic Conditions.* London: Brompton Hospital, 1960.

34. Ingram, R., Schilder, D.   Effect of pursed lips expiration on the pulmonary pressure flow relationship in obstructive lung disease. *Am. Rev. Respir. Dis.* 96:381, 1967.

35. Mueller, R., Petty, T.L., Filley, G.F., et al.   Ventilation and arterial blood gas changes induced by pursed lip breathing. *J. Appl. Physiol.* 28(6):784, 1970.

36. Motley, H.   The effects of slow deep breathing and the blood gas exchange within emphysema. *Am. Rev. Respir. Dis.* 88:485, 1963.

37. Paul, G., Eldridge, F., Mitchell, J., Fiene, T.   Some effects of slowing respiration rate in chronic emphysema and bronchitis. *J. Appl. Physiol.* 21(3):877, 1966.

38. Pfeiffer, V., Pfeiffer, A.   Breathing patterns and gas mixing. *Phys. Ther.* 44(5):331, 1964.

39. Guthrie, A., Petty, T.   Improved exercise tolerance in patients with chronic airway obstruction. *Phys. Ther.* 50(9):1333, 1970.

40. Leith, D., Bradley, M.   Ventilatory muscle strength and endurance training. *J. Appl. Physiol.* 41(4):508, 1976.

41. Keens, T.G., Krastins, I.R.B., Wannamaker, E.M., et al.   Ventilatory muscle endurance training in normal subjects and patients with cystic fibrosis. *Am. Rev. Respir. Dis.* 116:853, 1977.

42. Asher, M.I., Pardy, R.L., Coates, A.L., et al.   The effects of inspiratory muscle training in patients with cystic fibrosis. *Am. Rev. Respir. Dis.* 126:855, 1982.

43. Pardy, R.L., Rivington, R.N., Despas, P.J., Macklem, P.T.   Inspiratory muscle training compared with physiotherapy in patients with CAL. *Am. Rev. Respir. Dis.* 123:421, 1981.

44. Pardy, R.L., Rivington, R.N., Despas, P.J., Macklem, P.T.   The effects of inspiratory muscle training on exercise performance in CAL. *Am. Rev. Respir. Dis.* 123:426, 1981.

45. Belman, M.J., Mittman, C.   Ventilatory muscle training improves exercise capacity in chronic obstructive pulmonary disease patients. *Am. Rev. Respir. Dis.* 121:273, 1980.

46. Belman, M.J., Kendregan, B.   Physical training fails to improve ventilatory muscle endurance in patients with chronic obstructive pulmonary disease. *Chest* 81(4):440, 1982.

47. Casciari, R.J., Fairshter, R.D., Harrison, A., et al.   Effects of breathing retraining in patients with chronic obstructive pulmonary disease. *Chest* 79(4):393, 1981.

48. Astrand, P., Rodahl, K.   *Textbook of Work Physiology.* New York: McGraw-Hill, 1977.

49. Barach, A.L., Bickerman, H.A., Beck, G.J.   Advances in the

treatment of non-tuberculous pulmonary disease. *Bull. N.Y. Acad. Med.* 28(6):353, 1952.

50. Miller, W.F., Taylor, H.F., Pierce, A.K. Rehabilitation of the disabled patient with chronic bronchitis and pulmonary emphysema. *Am. J. Public Health* 53(Suppl. 3):18, 1963.

51. Paez, P.N., Phillipson, E.A., Masangkay, M., Sproule, B.J. The physiologic basis of training patients with emphysema. *Am. Rev. Respir. Dis.* 95:944, 1967.

52. Woolf, C.R., Suero, J.T. Alterations in lung mechanics and gas exchange following training in chronic obstructive lung disease. *Dis. Chest* 55(1):37, 1969.

53. Bass, H., Whitcomb, J.F., Forman, R. Exercise training: therapy for patients with chronic obstructive pulmonary disease. *Chest* 57(2):116, 1970.

54. Laros, C.D., Swierenga, J. Rehabilitation program in patients with obstructive lung disease: proposition for the selection of the most promising candidates. *Respiration* 29:344, 1972.

55. Vyas, M.N., Banister, E.W., Morton, J.W., Grzybowski, S. Response to exercise in patients with chronic airway obstruction. *Am. Rev. Respir. Dis.* 103:390, 1971.

56. Smodlaka, V.R., Adamovich, D.R. Reconditioning of emphysema patients using interval training. *N.Y. State J. Med.* 74:951, 1974.

57. Alison, J.A., Samios, R., Anderson, S.D. Evaluation of exercise training patients with chronic airway obstruction. *Phys. Ther.* 61(9):1273, 1981.

58. Belman, M.J., Kendregan, B.A. Exercise training fails to increase skeletal muscle enzymes in patients with chronic obstructive pulmonary disease. *Am. Rev. Respir. Dis.* 123:256, 1981.

59. Belman, M.J., Wasserman, K. Exercise training and testing in patients with chronic obstructive pulmonary disease. *Basics Respir. Dis.* 10 (2):1, 1981.

60. Miller, W.F., Taylor, H.F., Jasper L. Exercise training in the rehabilitation of patients with severe respiratory insufficiency due to pulmonary emphysema: the role of oxygen breathing. *South. Med. J.* 55:1216, 1962.

61. Arora, N.S., Rochester, D.F. Respiratory muscle strength and maximal voluntary ventilation in undernourished patients. *Am. Rev. Respir. Dis.* 126:5, 1982.

62. Nield, M.A. The effect of health teaching on the anxiety level of patients with chronic obstructive pulmonary disease. *Nurs. Res.* 20:537, 1971.

63. Perry, J.A. Effectiveness of teaching in the rehabilitation of patients with chronic bronchitis and emphysema. *Nurs. Res.* 30(4):219, 1981.

V Biomechanical Considerations

13 Power Output at Different Areas in the Range of Motion

John A. Clayton, Ph.D

Production of muscular power often is identified as a crucial parameter for success in movement activities [1]. When observing sports events, we frequently are reminded by the commentators of the power displayed by the competing athletes. This observation of power output on the part of the performer is evaluated most often in terms of the entire movement. However, the importance of analyzing, and then optimizing, power output at various areas in the range of motion (ROM) has been afforded little attention.

It is possible that even the most successful athletes have serious deficiencies in power production at distinct areas in the ROM, but unless specifically tested for, it is unlikely that these deficiencies would be discovered. The purpose of the present study was to scrutinize power production at distinctly different areas in the ROM for the bench press, which is one of the most widely used weight training exercises for the upper body.

Methods

Twenty-eight male university students who were members of a physical education weight training course volunteered to serve as subjects. Their mean age was 21.12 years, with a standard deviation of 1.38 years. After their informed consent to participate in the study was obtained, the subjects were tested for a maximal voluntary contraction (MVC) on the bench press station of a Universal Gym (Universal Gym Equipment Co., Cedar Rapids, Iowa).* International power lifting rules were followed as closely as possible in the determination of the MVC; test-retest reliability was 0.94, which is in close agreement with values previously reported [2].

In subsequent class sessions, power output on the bench press was obtained at a loading of 50 percent of the subject's MVC. Power output (P) was quantified through the use of the universal formula, $P = w/t$, where work (w) was the product of the weight and distance moved, and time (t) for the movement was measured via two Lafayette digital clock-counters (Lafayette Instrument Co., Lafayette, Ind.) which provided values to the

---

*See J.P. O'Shea, *Scientific Principles and Methods of Strength Fitness*. Reading, Mass.: Addison-Wesley, 1976, p. 183.

nearest millisecond. Microswitches were mounted on a vertical rod and positioned so that both clocks would start at the beginning of the movement. As the individual moved through the ROM, activation of the two remaining switches stopped one of the clocks when the halfway point was reached and the other at the end of the designated ROM.

Power was ascertained for the following conditions: (1) for a single repetition through the total range of motion (TROM) of 46 cm; (2) for the first 23 cm of the single repetition (ROM$_1$); (3) for the second 23 cm of the single repetition (ROM$_2$); and, (4) for a short range of motion (SROM) that started at the 23-cm point and terminated at the 46-cm distance. During the first testing session, the subjects were administered four consecutive trials through the TROM, resting for 30 seconds between trials. The criterion score was the mean of the four trials. Two days later, during the next class session, all subjects were given four consecutive trials through the SROM. Again, the intertrial rest period was 30 seconds and the mean score was taken as the criterion. Test-retest reliability for power output in the various conditions ranged from 0.91 to 0.93.

Results and Discussion

Several one-way analyses of variance were conducted to determine whether there were any significant differences for power output between the various conditions of interest. Table 13-1 shows that all comparisons made were statistically significant ($p < 0.001$). The indication is that movement condition is a major factor in the generation of power.

Figure 13-1 displays the means and standard deviations for power output. Inspection of this figure clearly shows that the greatest amount of power can be produced in the ROM$_2$ condition and, in descending order, in the SROM and ROM$_1$ conditions. The TROM values are included mainly for reference purposes.

There is nothing very surprising or unexpected in the mean values of the results. One would expect that the most power would be produced in the ROM$_2$, since the weight is already in motion and the inertia present with dead weight has been overcome. The situation is analogous to giving a sprinter a running start.

Table 13-1
F Ratios for One-Way Analysis of Variance Between Movement Conditions[a]

Condition	ROM$_2$	SROM
ROM$_1$	59.7	15.6
ROM$_2$		20.2

[a]All ratios are significant.

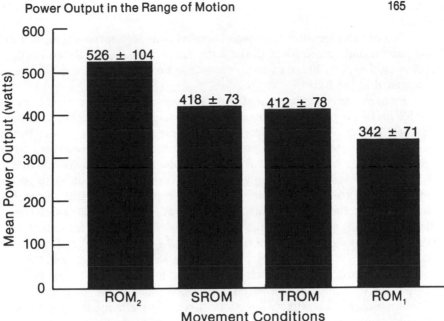

Figure 13-1. Mean power output (in watts; ±S.D.) for movement conditions.

The SROM and ROM$_1$ are similar in that both movements begin from a stop position and both movements cover a distance of 23 cm. However, they move through different areas in the ROM. The ROM$_1$ started with the bar at approximately chest level, and power was calculated for the first 23 cm. The SROM started at the point where the ROM$_1$ ended, and power was calculated for a 23-cm movement which ended approximately 46 cm above the chest.

The identical musculature will be used in completing these movements, but certain muscles may be able to contribute more (or less) to a given movement condition because of the particular length-tension relationship, force velocity situation, or the mechanical advantage available. Those individuals who are familiar with the bench press are well aware that the inability to complete the exercise is generally the result of being unable to move the bar past some specific point in the first half of the ROM, usually a point close to the chest. Likewise, a relatively common overload training technique is to perform partial repetitions on the bench press. This involves loading the bar with considerably more weight than the individual can handle through the full ROM; then the weight is lowered from a position of full extension of the arms toward the chest. In most cases the weight will not be lowered more than half of the way down and then it is pressed back to the position of full extension. The typical observation is that the trainee can exert substantially more force in the latter half of the ROM. Based on this, one would expect that greater power would be produced in the SROM as compared to the ROM_1.

Perhaps the most meaningful and interesting findings of the study reside in the analysis of power output for certain individuals. For example, Subject 21 was a varsity athlete, the strongest of the group on the bench press, and the second most powerful over the TROM. However, comparisons of his power outputs at ROM_1, ROM_2, and SROM are enlightening. On the average, the group was able to produce 24 percent more power in the SROM compared to the ROM_1, but Subject 21 generated 14 percent less power in the SROM. This placed him at -2.11 standard deviations from the group mean. Also, the group displayed 55 percent more power in the ROM_2 condition as compared to the ROM_1 condition; but Subject 21 created only 19 percent more power in the ROM_2, which placed him at -1.63 standard deviations below the group average. Therefore, in both conditions (i.e., SROM compared with ROM_1, and ROM_1 compared with ROM_2), Subject 21 ranked lowest in these relative comparisons. Such a finding suggests a real problem in power production during the second half of the ROM, independent of the movement condition.

Subject 28 was very near the mean for generating more power in the ROM_2 compared to the ROM_1 but was 2.34 standard deviations above the mean in his ability to produce more power for the SROM versus the ROM_1. In itself, this suggests a substantial capacity to create more power when starting at a higher point in the ROM. However, it was somewhat surprising to find that he actually produced 5 percent less power in the ROM_2, in contrast to the SROM condition. In the latter case, the bar was moved through the same ROM, but the subject put out less power when he had a moving start.

Analysis of the data for both of these trainees indicates atypical performance decrements for power production in at least one condition for the latter half of the ROM. These results may be due to different mechanisms. This relative inability to produce power may occur because of a specific weakness of the contributing musculature at that area in the ROM, or it may come about via an inhibitory effect of the nervous system as the end of the ROM is approached.

Breaking down a movement into specific areas of the ROM helps to identify more precisely what is happening. From the additional information, custom training programs may be formulated. Subject 21 might well have benefited from a weight training regimen that placed more emphasis on the second half of the ROM for the bench press or, perhaps, from special exercises that isolated the musculature that contributes most to motion in the latter part of the ROM. In contrast, Subject 28 could possibly have improved his ROM$_2$ performance through training techniques that accentuated extension (disinhibition).

Conclusion

The capacity to generate power on the bench press will differ depending on the movement condition. Because of varying mechanical and physiologic relationships, the amount of power that a muscle (or muscle group) may contribute to a movement is likely to fluctuate as the ROM is traversed. Power output may also be less than maximal if premature termination (through inhibition) of a movement occurs. Analysis of power production for the full ROM of a movement may help in identifying a specific area in the ROM for which an athlete's power production is less than optimal.

References

1. Wilmore, J.H. *Athletic Training and Physical Fitness*. Boston: Allyn and Bacon, 1976, p. 67.
2. Berger, R.A., Hardage, B. Effect of maximum loads for each of ten repetitions on strength development. *Res. Q.* 38:715–718, 1967.

14 Sculling: An Electromyographic Analysis

Jonathan S. Herland, B.S.

Any sport in which one engages competitively is performed best if it can be practiced at all times of the year. A problem sometimes arises in a sport such as sculling which cannot be performed under all weather conditions or through all seasons. For such sports it is clearly advantageous to perform a substitute activity that closely resembles the muscle recruitment pattern while simultaneously duplicating the intensity of the activity. The present study is aimed at identifying a suitable substitute activity for sculling. Therefore, an electromyographic (EMG) analysis was performed in order to determine the pattern of muscle recruitment during sculling. Comparisons are then made with muscle recruitment patterns of other activities [1, 2].

Materials

Pregelled, disposable, Premie silver-silverchloride electrocardiograph electrodes (Consolidated Medical Equipment, Inc., Utica, N.Y.), and three battery-powered amplifiers (10 × voltage gain) with a 1-second timing diode were used. Amplifiers were equipped with shielded cable leads to the recorders and to the electrodes. Also used were three battery-powered cassette recorders with magnetic tapes, a single gig with oars, and a polygraph recorder (Grass Instrument Co., Quincy, Mass.).

Protocol

After building and testing amplifiers to be certain of the accurate recoverability of the EMG signals, signals from the following muscles were successfully recorded while sculling: left vastus lateralis, left gluteus maximus, left rectus femoris, left gastrocnemius (lateral head), left tibialis anterior, right

Dr. Sheldon Simon of the Children's Hospital Medical Center, Boston, Massachusetts, is gratefully acknowledged for his encouragement and for providing use of his laboratory facilities. The author also wishes to thank especially Lance Jackson of the Gait Laboratory, Children's Hospital Medical Center, for his electronics expertise and limitless patience, without which it would have been impossible to collect any sculling data. The author also would like to thank Dr. Ernest Gervino of Beth Israel Hospital, Boston, for his assistance in collecting data, his practical suggestions, and his constant encouragement.

vastus lateralis, left adductor magnus, right vastus medialis, and left rectus abdominis. The size of the boat limited the number of recorders that could fit in it and so limited the number of muscles that could be monitored simultaneously. Therefore, it was decided that four trials, recording three muscles each, would be the most reasonable way of obtaining the desired data. The vastus lateralis was chosen as the reference muscle for two reasons: First, it generates a clear, strong, phasic signal, and second, its recruitment can indicate only one action—extension of the knee (or possibly stabilization of flexion, but this did not appear to occur).

Sculling was performed at 24 to 26 strokes per minute into a stiff but steady head wind at the highest controllable pressure (i.e., nearly full power). A special effort was made to be as consistent as possible in style from trial to trial. The recorded signals were located on the tapes with an oscilloscope and were recovered by the chart printer. Identification of the trials was accomplished by turning the amplifier on and off in a distinctive pattern a few moments before the start of each sculling trial. Synchronization of the chart strips was achieved by counting the 1-second timing spikes generated by the diode which was built into the amplifiers.

Results

Figure 14–1 shows a synthesis of the temporal pattern of recruitment of all nine muscles that were monitored. For a typical stroke in each trial, the duration of each signal was carefully measured and the beginning and end of each muscle's contraction was represented as a percentage of a stroke cycle. (Because the stroke rates of each trial could not possibly be identical, and because the tape recorders did not record at exactly the same rate, this was the only reasonable way to present the data.) It was decided arbitrarily that the stroke cycle began at the very beginning of electrical activity in the left vastus lateralis and ended at the beginning of the next period of electrical activity in the same muscle.

Discussion

It would be useful to compare recruitment patterns of certain muscles in sculling to those in walking [1], climbing stairs [2], and descending stairs [2]. Attention will first be focused on the quadriceps muscle group, because in rowing, more force is developed here than in any other muscle group [3]. The walking study examined the vastus lateralis and vastus medialis muscles (Figure 14–2). In walking, the vastus lateralis muscle showed electrical activity from prior to heel strike to shortly after, whereas the vastus medialis

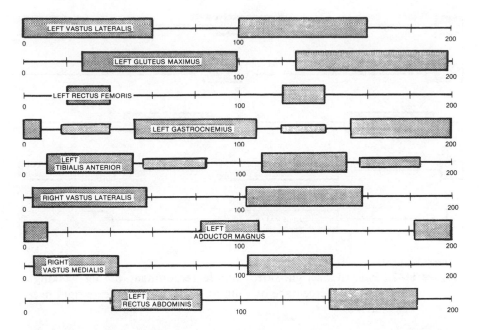

Figure 14-1. Temporal pattern of recruitment of nine muscles monitored electromyographically during sculling. Scale is percentage of a stroke cycle.

muscle is recruited from exactly at heel strike to shortly after the vastus lateralis becomes electrically silent. The sculling study indicated that the vastus lateralis and vastus medialis were recruited identically, with the vastus lateralis actually showing a longer period of electrical activity than the vastus medialis. These results are consistent with the hypothesis that the vastus lateralis is more of a "workhorse" muscle at the knee joint than is the vastus medialis. During walking, the vastus medialis is not required to help stabilize the knee until the weight of the entire body is brought to bear on the joint. During sculling, however, the resistive forces are relatively greater at the beginning of the "leg drive" (extension at both the knees and at the hips)—hence, the need to bring to bear the contractile power of more of the available muscle tissue. Near the end of the leg drive phase, when the boat speed is higher and therefore resistance to knee extension is lower, only the vastus lateralis (among the three superficial heads of the quadriceps) is needed to generate contractile power for continuing the extension of the knee.

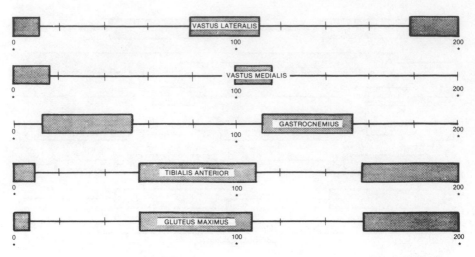

Source: Hardt [1], pp. 151, 155.

Figure 14–2. Pattern of right-sided muscle recruitment during walking. Scale is percentage of walking cycle. Stars indicate right heel strike.

The stair climbing and descending study examined the vastus medialis and rectus femoris muscles [2]. During stair climbing (Figure 14–3), both muscles simultaneously became electrically active at foot contact and electrically silent almost simultaneously when knee flexion was reduced to approximately 35 to 40 degrees. Because knee extension continued to approximately 5 to 10 degrees of flexion, one can infer that the rest of the quadriceps group was contracting to accomplish this. This is consistent with the finding during stair climbing, the highest moment (in Newton-meters) about the knee joint occurred shortly after the vastus medialis and rectus femoris became electrically active. In sculling, when acceleration of the boat is the greatest (during the middle of the leg drive phase) [4], one sees electrical activity in all three superficial heads of the quadriceps muscle group.

During stair descent, recruitment was considerably different, as was the action [2]. Because the action is one of resisting knee flexion rather than one of actually extending the knee, a different pattern of electrical activity might be expected, as is shown in Figure 14–4.

An examination of the gastrocnemius-tibialis anterior muscle complex for all four activities reveals that their electrical activities are in opposition with one another (as one would have expected). In addition, in the three propulsive activities (stair climbing, walking, sculling) the gastrocnemius muscle is recruited either at, or shortly before, turnoff for the vastus medialis muscle. In stair descent, the gastrocnemius is active only very briefly,

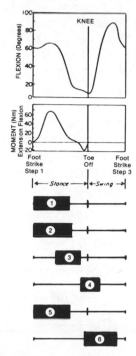

Source: Andriacchi et al. [2], p. 750.
Figure 14-3. Saggital plane flexion-extension movements of the knee; moments about the knee; and phasic activities of knee and ankle muscles in one limb of a subject ascending stairs. 1 = vastus medialis; 2 = rectus femoris; 3 = gastrocnemius; 4 = tibialis anterior; 5 = soleus; 6 = biceps femoris.

so it is difficult to draw a conclusion about its role. This would indicate that plantar flexion does not begin in any of the three propulsive activities until knee extension is either complete or nearly complete (as shown in Figure 14-3). This agrees with Williams's [3] theories on sequential recruitment of the lower-limb muscles during rowing, in which he states that these muscles are recruited in order from most powerful and slowest to least powerful and fastest—that is, hip extensors, knee extensors, plantar flexors, and digit flexors, respectively. What is interesting and unique about sculling is the biphasic contractile activity of both the gastrocnemius and tibialis anterior muscles, with the secondary phase of each appearing to be approximately one-half the electrical amplitude of the primary phase and occuring at approximately the same time as the primary contractile activity of the antagonistic muscle, as shown in Figure 14-1. These secondary contractions

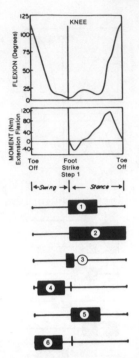

Source: Andriacchi et al. [2], p. 751.

Figure 14-4. Sagittal plane flexion-extension movements of the knee; moments about the knee; and phasic activities of knee and ankle muscles in one limb of a subject descending stairs. 1 = vastus medialis; 2 = rectus femoris; 3 = gastrocnemius; 4 = tibialis anterior; 5 = soleus; 6 = biceps femoris.

may be occurring to help stabilize the ankle during the primary contraction of the antagonist.

The strong and phasic electrical activity of the superficial part of the adductor magnus muscle (adductor portion) during sculling, as shown in Figure 14-1, was unexpected but suggests either a component of thigh adduction occurring ahead of knee extension or active assistance of hip flexion at the termination of the recovery phase of sculling. The rectus abdominis muscle also shows strong and phasic electrical activity (Figure 14-1), with initiation and termination of the signal occurring slightly ahead of those for the gastrocnemius muscle. This would indicate a stabilization of back extension occurring (and probably necessary only) after the back has passed the vertical position. This electrical activity would continue through the recovery phase (flexion occuring at the hip) until the very beginning of the propulsive phase, as indicated by the recruitment of the adductor magnus muscle at nearly the precise instant that the rectus abdominis muscle is allowed to relax.

The gluteus maximus muscle was monitored in the walking and sculling studies, but in both cases, the signals produced were of very poor quality.

Comments

Recruitment of quadriceps muscles during the propulsive phase of sculling is strikingly similar to that of the same muscles during the propulsive phase of stair climbing. Although walking is not nearly as strenuous as sculling, the overall (lower-limb) muscle recruitment is similar enough to help tone a sculler's propulsive muscles. The recruitment pattern from the stair descent study is different enough from sculling that stair descent would be a poor training substitute. Therefore, stair climbing is recommended (in the absence of any knee injury) as the closest training substitute for sculling.

The techniques employed in this study probably are applicable for EMG recording of activities that do not lend themselves easily to the use of conventional EMG equipment. An extra advantage of these techniques is the creation of a permanent record of all signals for subsequent analysis. This technique could be improved by multiplexing the signals from several muscles onto one tape, thereby eliminating the tedious process of synchronizing three or more chart tapes from the same recording trial. Recording signals from identical muscles in a two-, four-, or eight-oared crew could provide information about how compatibly crew members are sculling or rowing. Coordination with cinematographic data is clearly the next step in obtaining definitive kinesiologic information.

References

1. Hardt, D.E.   A Minimum Energy Solution for Muscle Force Control During Walking. Ph.D. diss., Massachusetts Institute of Technology, 1979.

2. Andriacchi, T.P., Andersson, G.B.J., Fermier, R.W.   A study of lower limb mechanics during stair climbing. *J. Bone Joint Surg.* [Am.] 62 A(5):749–57, 1980.

3. Williams, J.G.P. (ed.)   *Rowing: A Scientific Approach*. Cranbury, N.J.: A.S. Barnes, 1967, pp. 81–109.

4. Martin, T.P., Bernfeld, J.   Quantification in rowing. *The Oarsman*. 12(2):20–24, 1980.

VI Team Sports Injury Prevention and Rehabilitation

15 Injury Prevention and Rehabilitation in Baseball

Robert C. Cantu, M.D.

Baseball is primarily a noncontact sport. Therefore, it is not surprising that it is one of the safest schoolboy sports. Football, wrestling, hockey, and basketball account for most schoolboy sports injuries, whereas track, tennis, and baseball can be found at the other end of the spectrum. However, baseball alone among these safest sports is associated with some risk (albeit minimal) for life-threatening injury as a result of a thrown or batted ball striking a player's head. This chapter addresses the potential injuries in baseball—specifically, shoulder and elbow injuries—their prevention, and rehabilitation in the event of an injury.

Table 15-1 shows the Children's Hospital Medical Center's Division of Sports Medicine's baseball injury experience through June 1982. Injuries to the knee accounted for 41 percent of patients seen, with chondromalacia patellae and internal derangements the most frequent diagnoses, and injuries to the ankle and foot were present in 13 percent of patients. Shoulder and elbow injuries, which were more expected, were seen in only 7 percent of patients each. The structures of the body that were injured most often in baseball are outlined in Table 15-2. Muscle, tendon, or ligament injuries were the most common (38%), followed by bone (31%) and cartilage (25%) injuries.

These figures are somewhat slanted because they represent the most serious injuries, exclusive of craniofacial trauma which would be treated acutely. They also do not include the most common minor baseball injuries, including abrasions, contusions, and minor sprains and strains for which medical help beyond the trainer is not sought.

Pitchers and catchers are the players most vulnerable to injury. Owing to the nature of these positions, the shoulder and elbow are the most often injured areas of the body, as most studies of baseball players indicate [1-7]. It must be remembered that, although the upper extremity is a critical end-organ in the act of throwing, the coordination and balance of the rest of the body is vital. An inflamed great toe or low back pain may disrupt the athlete's body's muscular rhythm and alter throwing biomechanics, leading to shoulder injury.

Fimrite [8] popularized the "Dizzy Dean syndrome," the situation of creating a second injury by favoring a prior one. Dizzy Dean, an overpower-

The author wishes to thank Mr. Victor Quale for his help with the artwork used in this chapter.

Table 15-1
Children's Hospital Medical Center (Boston) Division of Sports Medicine
Baseball Injury Experience Through June 1982: Location of Injury

Location	No.	% Total
Knee	90	41
Ankle or foot	29	13
Shoulder	16	7
Elbow	15	7
Back	15	7
Hip	6	3
Hand	4	2
Miscellaneous other	44	20
Total	219	100

ing right-handed pitcher for the St. Louis Cardinals in the 1930s, was struck on the left foot by a line drive, suffering a broken big toe in the 1937 all-star game. Two weeks later, wearing a splint and an oversized shoe, he attempted to return to pitching. Favoring his injured toe altered Dean's natural pitching motion and led to a shoulder injury, which eventually was diagnosed as an inflammation of the deltoid muscle at its insertion on the humerus. This 30-plus ball game winner was to win only 16 games before his premature retirement 4 years later. Smokey Joe Wood, another baseball pitcher, suffered a similar fate. Known for his fastball and a winner of 34 games in 1912, Wood fell fielding a ground ball in the spring of 1913, sustaining a fractured thumb on his pitching hand. He, too, attempted to return to pitching too soon and, with an altered delivery, incurred a shoulder injury that cut short his career.

Shoulder Injuries

Anatomy of the Shoulder

The shoulder is a complex region consisting of the glenohumeral joint, its static capsular support (Fig. 15-1), and the dynamic muscle groups that control the motion of the shoulder girdle (Figs. 15-2, 15-3). The shoulder has the widest range of motion of any joint in the body. Normal function at the sternoclavicular joint, the acromioclavicular joint, and along the scapular thoracic plane are essential for full activity of the upper extremity.

The capsule of the shoulder joint lends static support to the glenohumeral joint. The rotator cuff muscles—the subscapularis anteriorly, the supraspinatus superiorly, and the infraspinatus and teres minor posteriorly—blend with the capsule and attach into the proximal humerus. The

Table 15-2
Children's Hospital Medical Center (Boston) Division of Sports Medicine Baseball Injury Experience Through June 1982: Structure Injured

Body Structure	No.	% Total
Muscle, tendon, or ligament	83	38
Bone	68	31
Cartilage	55	25
Nerve	3	1
Other	10	5

biceps tendon extends from the glenoid cavity through the joint superiorly and into the bicipital groove between the greater and lesser tuberosities of the humerus.

Overuse Syndromes

The painful "pitcher's shoulder" has plagued participants, trainers, and physicians of throwing sports teams for years, and now similar chronic overuse syndromes involving the shoulder are seen frequently among recreational and competitive swimmers [9–11] and tennis enthusiasts [12]. In-

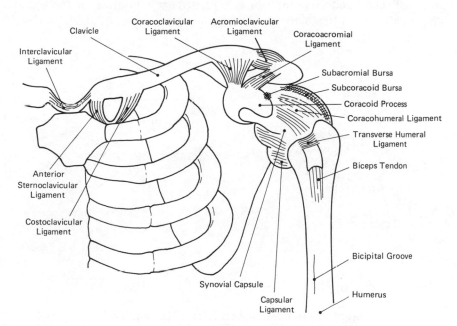

Figure 15-1. Bones, ligaments, capsule, and bursae of the shoulder.

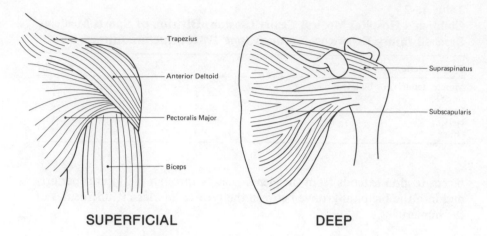

Figure 15-2. Anterior muscles of the shoulder.

sidious in onset and only annoying in their initial stages, these syndromes may increase relentlessly in intensity and severity and eventually may totally disable the athlete.

An *overuse syndrome* is defined as a chronic inflammatory condition caused by repeated microtrauma from a repetitious activity. Blazina [13] originally classified these injuries as (1) first-degree injuries, or those that cause pain only after activity, (2) second-degree injuries, which produce

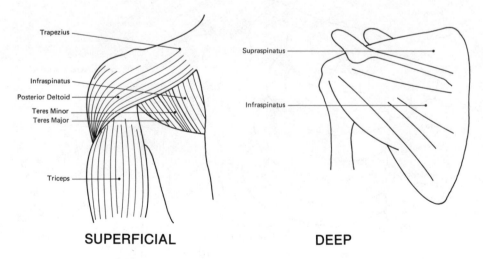

Figure 15-3. Posterior muscles of the shoulder.

pain during participation and after it, but not of sufficient intensity to interfere with performance, and (3) third-degree injuries, which result in disabling pain both during and after participation.

The Mechanism of Throwing. To appreciate the spectrum of injuries that may occur in throwing, one must comprehend the mechanism of this strenuous activity. Tullos [14–16] has classified the phases of throwing and pointed out those structures that participate in each step.

During the intial cocking motion (Fig. 15–4), the arm is brought back into abduction, extension, and external rotation. Consequently, the middle and posterior aspects of the deltoid muscle are functioning, as are the infraspinatus and teres minor, to produce rotation. The trapezius and rhomboid muscles contribute to scapular elevation and adduction. During the cocking stage, the posterior capsule is relaxed, whereas the anterior capsule, subscapularis, and pectoral muscles are passively elongating.

The next stage of throwing consists of the acceleration phase, in which the arm begins to move forward again, often preceded by a forward rotation of the trunk. During this activity, the anterior muscle groups, particularly the subscapularis, pectoral, and anterior deltoid muscles, are contracting while still lengthening eccentrically. The biceps muscle also may contract, increasing tension on the tendon within the bicipital groove, which is externally rotated. It is during this early part of the acceleration phase that the anterior capsule is particularly stretched. As the arm comes forward into the final follow-through position, the posterior capsule and external rotator muscles are relaxed and passively stretched.

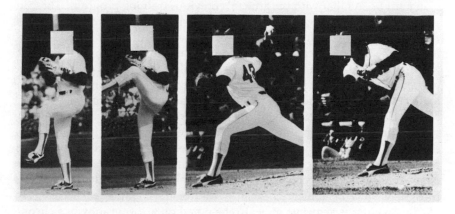

Source: R.C. Cantu, *Sports Medicine in Primary Care.* Lexington, Mass.: The Collamore Press, 1982, p. 179.

Figure 15–4. Phases of throwing: (A) windup; (B) cocking; (C) acceleration; and (D) follow-through.

Lesions that can occur during throwing include:

1. Attenuation of the anterior capsular ligaments, allowing the humeral head to sublux or even dislocate
2. Sudden contractions of the subscapularis and pectoral muscles, producing tears or rupture of these muscular tendinous units
3. Impingement anteriorly around the coracoid process and also posteriorly as the humeral head abuts on the glenoid cavity
4. Abutment of the biceps tendon and supraspinus tendon on the acromion and coracoacromial ligament, producing impingement syndromes
5. Small tears in the rotator cuff muscles as well as chronic subdeltoid bursitis as a result of these repeated impingements
6. Hypertrophic bony changes along the inferior aspect of the glenoid cavity and chronic subluxation of the biceps tendon from its groove
7. Chronic degenerative changes at the acromioclavicular joint, producing pain felt over the top of the shoulder and radiating both anteriorly and posteriorly

Clearly, the throwing mechanism is very complex and can cause symptoms and injuries in numerous areas. A great deal of diligence is required in questioning and examining patients with apparent throwing injuries to determine the site of the pathology.

Diagnosis. A careful history is perhaps the most important step in making the diagnosis of overuse syndromes. A previous history of shoulder subluxation or an acromioclavicular joint separation should be pursued. The clinician must be familiar with the athlete's previous training program. These injuries frequently are seen early in the season and often during periods of double-session workouts. Repeated examinations often are necessary to localize the site of the tenderness and particularly to detect relative weaknesses in the rotator muscle groups. A complete neurologic examination is needed to rule out cervical radiculitis, entrapment of the suprascapular or axillary nerves, and thoracic outlet syndromes. Vascular problems in the subclavian and brachial systems must also be considered.

Routine roentgenograms, including the Westpoint view to demonstrate the glenoid cavity should be obtained. Exostoses along the anterior and inferior aspects of the glenoid cavity may require special views. Degenerative changes at the acromioclavicular joint must also be ruled out. Shoulder arthrograms may be indicated when a rotator cuff tear is suspected (Fig. 15-5). An enlarged capsule may also be noted on arthrography in a chronic subluxing shoulder. Jackson [3] has pointed out that chronic impingement syndromes produce thickening and contraction of the subdeltoid bursa. He has performed bursagrams which nicely illustrate this problem. These addi-

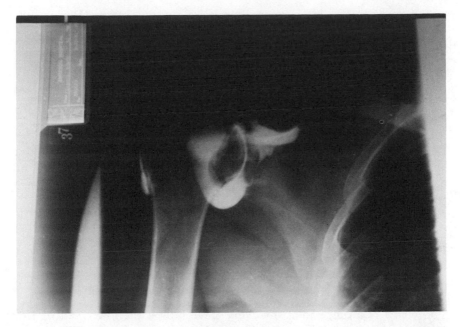

Figure 15-5. Tear in rotator cuff muscle as shown on shoulder arthrogram.

tional x-ray studies should be done only after a careful examination has been performed to determine the exact site of tenderness, the arc of motion that produces pain, and the presence of any specific weakness.

Treatment. Treatment of these overuse syndromes is directed at reducing inflammation and altering training and performance techniques to prevent recurrence. The first-degree and second-degree injuries, which produce pain primarily after participation and are not disabling, should be treated promptly to prevent their progression. Proper warm-up prior to sports participation and then ice applied to the shoulder following competition may help to relieve the inflammatory changes. Oral antiinflammatory agents such as aspirin or one of the other nonsteroidal medications often are helpful. Reducing the amount of time spent throwing may help to control the pain. It is essential that the patient review the problem with the coach, since minor changes in technique, such as the amount of elevation of the arm in throwing, may be necessary. Because these injuries frequently lead to contracture and muscle weakness, it is essential to seek these problems out and correct them with flexibility exercises and specific strengthening programs. The isokinetic machines are very helpful in detecting relative weaknesses about the shoulder.

The third-degree injuries usually require a period of rest. During this time, conditioning programs for the other areas of the body may be continued. Local injections of steroids into the involved areas have been helpful in some cases. However, it must be remembered that these injections produce local tissue necrosis and weaken the structures for at least 2 weeks [17]. During that time, no vigorous sports participation should be undertaken. Other modalities can be used to reduce inflammation, especially ultrasonic radiation and diathermy. Recurrence of these injuries is very common, and so the participant must have full *range of motion, equal strength,* and be *pain-free* before returning to competition. Since both coordination and shoulder endurance are essential in baseball, it is important to progress the rehabilitation program slowly to avoid future difficulties.

Elbow Injuries

Anatomy of the Elbow

The elbow is a hinge joint involving three bones: the lower end of the humerus, the upper end of the radius, and the olecranon and coronoid processes of the ulna (Figs. 15-6, 15-7). The radius can rotate around the ulna, allowing for supination and pronation of the forearm. The annular, ulnar, and radial collateral ligaments and articular capsule maintain joint stability.

Elbow Sprain

Treatment of an elbow sprain is similar to that of the shoulder. There is initial application of ice for the first 12 to 24 hours, and heat thereafter. The elbow is immobilized in a sling for 7 or more days until all pain on motion has ceased. Oral antiinflammatory medications—aspirin, indomethacin (Indocin), phenylbutazone (Butazolidin), ibuprofen (Motrin), tolmetin sodium (Tolectin), or sulindac (Clinoril)—may be used during this period. Thereafter, active flexion, extension, supination, and pronation exercises are given to the patient, and return to competition is dependent on the return of strength in the injured arm equal to the noninjured side.

Overuse Syndromes

"Tennis elbow," an inflammation of the aponeurosis overlying the extensor carpi radialis and the extensor communis pollicis et indicis muscles, is

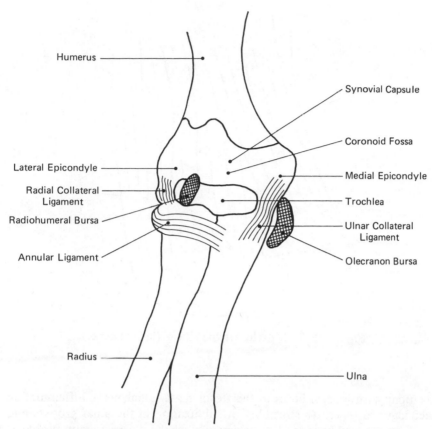

Figure 15–6. Bones, ligaments, capsule, and bursae of the elbow.

the most common overuse syndrome and is due to recurrent microtrauma at the elbow.

The second most common overuse elbow injury results from the act of throwing. As with the shoulder, the elbow may be injured commonly in throwing sports, swimming, and tennis, as the forces moving through the shoulder in the act of throwing or similar athletic motion are extended distally through the arm to the elbow. The acceleration and follow-through, the final phases of throwing, place tremendous stress on the elbow. The medial side of the elbow is stretched and the lateral side is compressed, as are the olecranon and distal humerus. In the follow-through motion, extreme compressive forces are generated in the concavity of the olecranon and its tip from the pull of the triceps tendon. Pathologic conditions result in these sites in athletes who engage in repetitive throwing motion (Fig. 15–8, 15–9).

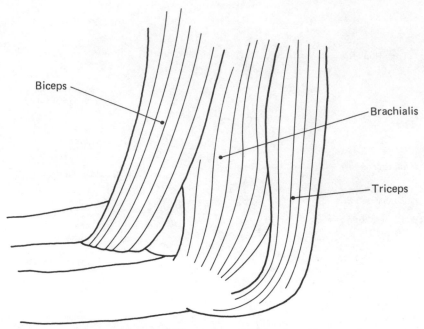

Figure 15-7. Muscles of the elbow (lateral aspect).

Bony avulsions, injuries to the flexor mass, ulnar nerve inflammation secondary to repetitive stretching or subluxation in the ulnar groove, and spurs on the medial edge of the olecranon are the most common problems occurring on the medial side of the elbow from throwing. All these conditions must be considered in the differential diagnosis. In the young athlete, frank avulsion of the medial epicondyle also must be considered.

The compressive forces on the lateral side of the elbow between the radial head and the capitulum humeri result in a shearing action on the radiohumeral joint, resulting in damage to the articular cartilage, with progressive fragmentation and formation of intraarticular loose bodies. In the preadolescent athlete, a focal avascular necrosis called *Panner's disease* may be identified in the capitulum humeri. Furthermore, the compressive force of the traction pull of the triceps impacts the tip of the olecranon against the olecranon fossa of the humerus and may result in articular damage, fragmentation, and loose body formation.

In the skeletally immature athlete with open epiphyses, compressive lateral forces may lead to abnormalities of growth, premature degeneration as in the adult, and long-term intraarticular deformity. "Little League elbow," the nonunion of a stress fracture through the olecranon growth

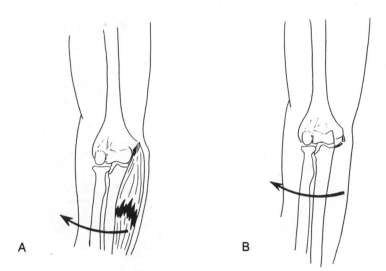

Source: R.C. Cantu, *Sports Medicine in Primary Care.* Lexington, Mass.: The Collamore Press, 1982, p. 184.

Figure 15–8. (A) Flexor muscle tears. (B) Medial collateral ligament rupture.

plate, is such an example. Although it is impossible to define, in terms of chronologic age, when a young athlete with open epiphyses and active growth potential should and should not pitch, as this is related to individual skeletal development and maturation, the Little League restrictions for limited pitching are strongly recommended. Clearly, the greater the number of innings pitched by a youth with open epiphyses, the more likely is that child to develop anatomic elbow impairment and ultimately to suffer restriction of an athletic career. The curveball and screwball, because of the snap supination involved in their performance, produce the greatest stress on the elbow, and so it is recommended that they be thrown only by the skeletally mature athlete. The medial epicondyle of the humerus is the last of the epiphyseal centers of the elbow to close, usually after age 14 years.

Treatment of Elbow Injuries

The treatment of any of the previously described throwing injuries to the elbow should involve orthopedic referral if any of the various bone pathologies are visible on roentgenography. If ulnar neuritis is present with numbness of the fifth finger and lateral half of the fourth finger, usually without intrinsic muscle weakness or atrophy in the early stages, neurosurgical referral is suggested.

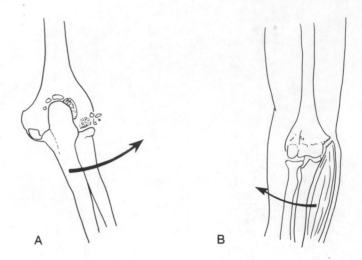

Source: R.C. Cantu, *Sports Medicine in Primary Care.* Lexington, Mass.: The Collamore Press, 1982, p. 185.

Figure 15-9. (A) Medial epicondylar avulsion fracture. (B) Ulnar traction spur and medial collateral ligament attenuation.

References

1. Bennett, G.E.   Shoulder and elbow lesions of the professional baseball pitcher. *J.A.M.A.* 117:510, 1941.

2. Bennett, G.E.   Shoulder and elbow lesions distinctive of baseball players. *Am. Surg.* 126:107, 1947.

3. Jackson, D.W.   Chronic rotator cuff impingement in the throwing athlete. *Am. J. Sports Med.* 4(6):231, 1976.

4. King, J.W., Brelsford, H.J., Tullos, H.S.   Analysis of the pitching arm of the professional baseball pitcher. *Clin. Orthop.* 67:116, 1969.

5. Lombardo, S.J., Jobe, R.W., Kerlan, R., et al.   Posterior shoulder lesions in throwing athletes. *Am. J. Sports Med.* 5:106, 1977.

6. Norwood, L.A., Jobe, F.W., et al.   Anterior shoulder pain in baseball pitchers. *Am. J. Sports Med.* 6(3):103, 1978.

7. Pappas, A.M.   Injuries of the upper extremities. In Vinger, P.F., Hoerner, E.F. (eds.), *Sports Medicine, The Unthwarted Epidemic.* Littleton, Mass.: PSG Publishing, 1981.

8. Fimrite, R.   Stress, strain, and pain. *Sports Illustrated,* August 14, 1978, pp. 30-43.

9. Kennedy, J.C., Hawkins, P.T.   Swimmer's shoulder. *Physician Sportsmed.* 2:35-38, 1974.

10. Kennedy, J.C., et al.   Orthopedic manifestations of swimming. *Am. J. Sports Med.* 6:309, 1978.

11. Richardson, A.B., Jobe, E.W., Collins, R.H.   The shoulder in competitive swimming. *Am. J. Sports Med.* 8(3):159, 1980.

12. Priest, J.D., Nagel, D.A.   Tennis shoulder. *Am. J. Sports Med.* 4(1):28, 1976.

13. Blazina, M.E.   Jumper's knee. *Orthop. Clin. North Am.* 4:665, 1973.

14. Barnes, D.A., Tullos, H.S.   An analysis of 100 symptomatic baseball players. *Am. J. Sports Med.* 6(2):62, 1978.

15. Tullos, H.S., King, J.W.   Lesions of the pitching arm in adolescents. *J.A.M.A.* 220:264-271, 1972.

16. Tullos, H.S., King, J.W.   Throwing mechanism in sports. *Orthop. Clin. North Am.* 4:709-720, 1973.

17. Kennedy, J.C., Willis, R.B.   The effects of local steroid injections on tendons: a biomechanical and microscopic correlative study. *Am. J. Sports Med.* 4:11-21, 1976.

16 Injury Prevention and Rehabilitation in Track

G. Richard Paul, M.D.

In this chapter, six injury patterns in runners are presented, and the clinical findings and treatment of each condition is described. Although each process is associated with its own unique findings and treatment, there are symptoms common in the development of all the conditions that suggest ways to prevent track-related injury.

Common Running Injuries

The six running injury patterns will be discussed in sequence, moving in a proximal-to-distal direction in the lower extremity. The conditions include:

1. Lateral patellar compression syndrome
2. Iliotibial band friction syndrome
3. Achilles tendinitis
4. Posterior tibial tendinitis
5. Plantar fasciitis
6. Stress fractures

Most of these are examples of overuse syndromes of the lower extremity.

Lateral Patellar Compression Syndrome

The lateral patellar compression syndrome is characterized by pain in the lateral aspect of the patellofemoral joint. Increased mileage, hard surfaces, hills or inclines, and interval workouts all have been cited as contributing factors in a runner's development of the condition. Contributing static deformities include hip internal rotation, internal rotation of the patella (characterized as "medial squint of the patella" by James [1]), varus deformity of either the knee or tibia, external tibial torsion, and excessive foot pronation. Each of these deformities compounds the compressive forces already existing on the patellofemoral articulation.

Treatment of the patellofemoral compression syndrome is simply rest. Rarely is surgery required [2]. Prophylaxis before the condition becomes consistently symptomatic and rehabilitation after the acute phase has resolved includes realignment of the lower extremities by the use of orthoses, quadriceps strengthening exercises (either isometric or limited terminal extension isotonic exercises), and a revision of the training program to eliminate the contributing factors.

Iliotibial Band Friction Syndrome

The iliotibial band is one of the major lateral stabilizers of the knee. It helps to rotate the tibia externally and thereby stabilize the knee at heel strike. The iliotibial band passes over the lateral femoral epicondyle, and it passes from back to front over the epicondyle as the knee goes from the flexed to extended position.

The iliotibial band friction syndrome is caused by excessive repeated contact between the iliotibial band and the lateral femoral epicondyle during flexion and extension of the knee. The result is either inflammation of the bursa overlying the lateral femoral epicondyle or direct irritation of the iliotibial band itself or the periosteum of the femoral epicondyle.

The syndrome usually develops because of training errors, primarily excessive distances covered or runs on downgrades, for which prolonged knee stabilization is required. Contributing static deformities include varus deformity of the knee, whereby excessive friction of the iliotibial band is applied against the femoral epicondyle, and a tight iliotibial band itself. Runners who consistently run on the same side of a pitched road develop the iliotibial band syndrome on the down-side leg because of the varus stress repeatedly applied to that knee.

Treatment for established iliotibial band friction syndrome consists of rest. The running program must be broken or stopped entirely. Walking with the knee in extension will minimize friction between the iliotibial band and the femoral epicondyle. Occasionally, nonsteroidal antiinflammatory medications or salicylates are needed to promote healing. On rare occasions, injection of the bursa is required.

Prophylactic treatment, once the acute process has resolved, includes exercises to stretch the iliotibial band and quadriceps strengthening exercises. Running should be resumed on the opposite slope of a pitched road, with the injured leg on the upgrade, and runs on downgrades, where heel strike and knee stabilization is prolonged, should be minimized.

Partial surgical release of the iliotibial band, effectively eliminating a portion of the band from sliding over the femoral epicondyle, has been described [3]. It must be advised with caution, however, for the iliotibial band is an important stabilizer of the knee at heel strike.

Achilles Tendinitis

Achilles tendinitis is by far the most common form of tendinitis seen in runners. The runner initially notes pain just above the heel counter, usually several hours after training, following which symptoms are present while running and usually at heel strike. Examination at this early stage may reveal crepitation or inflammation of the paratenon or even localized tenderness without a palpable defect in the tendon. Only later, following repeated episodes of acute tendinitis, can a defect or significant thickening of the paratenon be noted. Contributing factors frequently include a change in running surface or in training patterns, such as increased mileage, interval training, or hill running.

Puddu [4] has classified tendon injury into three categories:

1. *Tenosynovitis* or *tenovaginitis* is inflammation of only the paratenon, which may or may not be lined by synovium.
2. *Tendinitis* is injury or symptomatic degeneration of the tendon with resultant inflammatory reaction of the surrounding paratenon.
3. *Tendinosis* is asymptomatic tendon degeneration due to aging or accumulated microtrauma.

There are two potential causes of Achilles tendinitis, which falls into Puddu's second category. First, repeated loading of the musculotendinous unit may lead to muscle fatigue, reflex muscle spasm, and ultimately decreased flexibility. For example, the gastrocnemius muscle in distance runners must be relaxed to allow for heel strike. If it is tight from fatigue, the Achilles tendon then is subjected to increased loading. Runners with Achilles tendinitis are most symptomatic not at push-off but at heel strike, when the Achilles tendon is being stretched. Second, repetitive active loading of the musculotendinous unit may lead to collagen failure. This fatigue or stress failure of tendon is analogous to bone failure in stress fractures.

Treatment involves immediate rest of the tendon. This may include simply not running, the use of a heel lift, or even cast immobilization, depending on the severity of the acute process. Once the acute episode has resolved, a vigorous stretching program must be undertaken to restore full mobility to the Achilles tendon, followed thereafter by calf strengthening exercises and resumption of running on a controlled and graduated basis.

The hazards of steroids to tendon and articular cartilage are well known to orthopedists. Steroid injection rarely is indicated in the Achilles tendon. Steroid injections not only mask the symptoms, giving the runner a false sense of healing, but they actually inhibit tendon healing and directly decrease the tensile strength of tendons. Injections in the tendo calcaneus can result in permanent destruction of the tendon and, occasionally, in complete tendon rupture.

Posterior Tibial Tendinitis

The posterior tibial tendon is one of the major forefoot stabilizers, bringing the forefoot into plantar flexion and inversion and thereby stabilizing the forefoot against pronation during midstance and push-off. Posterior tibial tendinitis usually is seen at the beginning of a training program. Contributing factors include running on asphalt or concrete or even running on rough ground where excessive forefoot pronation-supination forces are applied. Forefoot pronation is the most common traumatic malalignment noted. Clinicians are cautioned to obtain radiographs of the foot or ankle to ascertain that a stress fracture of the distal tibia, medial malleolus, or tarsal navicular has not been overlooked.

Treatment is essentially the same as for Achilles tendinitis—appropriate rest or immobilization, followed by stretching and calf strengthening exercises. If there is excessive forefoot pronation, a flexible foot orthosis with a medial heel wedge will help prevent a recurrence of posterior tibial tendinitis.

Plantar Fasciitis

Plantar fasciitis, like the two tendinitis syndromes just described, is an injury of collagen fibers from repetitive overloading. The plantar fascia can be likened to a tension cable, spanning the length of the foot from the calcaneus to the metatarsals and thereby helping to maintain the longitudinal arch. Repetitive overloading of the foot results in a microscopic tear of the plantar fascia at its origin from the medial process of the calcaneus. It is seen far more commonly in distance runners than in sprinters [5], further indication that it represents repetitive overloading of the fascia. As pain becomes more constant and intense, the runner attempts to compensate by keeping his or her foot in a rather supinated or inverted position from the time of heel strike through toe push-off. The condition must be differentiated from the more unusual entitites of tarsal tunnel syndrome or plantar nerve entrapment.

Treatment consists of rest, since this is a fatigue failure of the plantar fascia. Adequate time must be allowed for proper repair of the collagen tissue. Steroid injections are not recommended, for reasons described under Achilles Tendinitis (p. 195). The use of a heel cup or a medial heel wedge will help prevent a recurrence, because it shields the plantar fascia and redistributes weight bearing so that stress on the plantar fascia is minimized.

If symptoms continue unremittingly for 4 to 6 months, partial surgical re-section of the plantar fascia is advised.

Stress Fractures

As the term aptly suggests, stress fractures are the result of repetitive overloading of a bone subjected to a stress for which it is unprepared. Here again, training errors are the significant factor. The bones cannot handle the repetitive overloading applied to them as a result of fatigued muscles unable to act properly as shock absorbers for the lower extremities. Similar fracture patterns occur in military recruits and athletes in a too-vigorous track training program. One observer has noted that stress fractures occur in three athletic animals—race dogs, race horses, and humans.

If the diagnosis is in doubt or immediate diagnosis is critical, a bone scan will help. The bone scan will be positive within 24 to 48 hours of fracture, well before a standard radiograph would confirm the diagnosis at 10 to 14 days. This is particularly helpful in dealing with a track athlete who must maintain his or her training program for a meet.

Treatment consists of rest until healing of the stress fracture is adequately mature. The specific treatment will vary with the particular fracture. Those in noncritical areas—the pelvis, fibula, metatarsals, or calcaneus—can be treated simply by refraining from running. Normal shoe wear may be continued. A longer interval of restricted activity, perhaps combined with a walking cast, is needed for stress fractures in moderately critical areas, such as the femoral and tibial midshafts. Those fractures at critical levels—the femoral neck or the proximal tibia—require protected weight bearing ambulation with crutches. Stress fractures in critical areas must be followed closely with periodic radiographs to be certain that displacement, particularly of a femoral neck fracture, does not develop.

Substitute sports are particularly helpful with stress fractures if an athlete wants to maintain the stretching and strengthening programs of the lower extremities but avoid the repetitive shock absorbing of running. Race walking, swimming, and bicycling all are appropriate, but it must be remembered that, although a substitute sport can maintain cardiovascular conditioning and lower-extremity tone, it will not maintain the precise muscle conditioning of running.

Injury Analysis

An analysis of all the conditions cited reveals certain recurring patterns; several common features are apparent.

First, *pain* occurred while running and increased while running. Second, symptoms developed with a *new training program*. The changes in the training program took one of three forms: (1) a new regimen, such as interval training or increased mileage; (2) a new route or training surface, such as inclines, pitches, or variations in surface grade; or (3) new equipment. A third common feature of all the conditions is that the *structures are at risk*. Bone, tendon, and fascia are not ready to handle the repetitive overloading suddenly demanded of them. Cardiovascular tone in humans, particularly in the younger athlete, can be developed more rapidly than the tensile strength and resiliency of muscle, tendon, or bone. In addition, whereas bone density and strength will improve with time and whereas muscles can be strengthened, the collagen fiber of tendon and fascia frequently will not respond to strengthening even when given adequate time. This is particularly true with the older runner.

The running conditions discussed above fall into three areas for analysis, effectively a triad of risk factors: (1) anatomic malalignment, (2) equipment failure, and (3) training errors. It is the third area that is the source of most problems and certainly the one area fully within our control. We can do little about anatomic malalignment, other than to recognize that foot orthoses can provide medial support of the heel and thereby decrease hindfoot eversion and forefoot pronation and, perhaps, reduce varus stress on the knee. We can replace or modify equipment to a degree. For example, we can certainly get new or proper shoes, if we cannot improve the surface of the high school track. Training errors, however, are entirely within our control, and it is here that we can have the greatest impact on injury prevention.

Injury Treatment or Prevention

Rest or Modification of the Routine

Pain is the body's signal that something is wrong. Unlike a contusion in football—a hip pointer or shoulder contusion, for instance—for which exercise through pain will help, pain that develops with running is a warning that trouble lies ahead. It is, in effect, a signal of excessive stress on the joint surfaces and bones and on the collagen tissue of tendons and fascia, and it cannot be ignored.

Accordingly, rest or a modification of the training routine is required, combined with a positive stretching and strengthening program. The distance traveled may be shortened, such as for lateral patellar compression syndrome. Running may be completely discontinued and alternate exercise programs of bicycling or swimming may be substituted, such as for tendinitis, plantar fasciitis, or stress fractures. Alternatively, the slope or pitch of the running surface may be varied, such as for the iliotibial band friction syndrome, or inclines may be limited, such as for lateral patellar compression syndrome.

Strengthening

A positive program of muscle strengthening of the lower extremities also is required. Whether this involves isometric, isotonic, or isokinetic strengthening depends on the specific condition. Isometric strengthening is required in situations where knee motion must be restricted, such as in the lateral patellar compression and iliotibial band friction syndromes. As the acute process subsides, progression to partial isotonic strengthening is advised. Isokinetic strengthening is perhaps best, using a variable force throughout muscle contraction so that a constant resistance to muscle contraction is applied. Isokinetic exercise permits strengthening of all muscle groups about the joint, both flexors and extensors, in the most dynamic fashion. Muscles must be allowed adequate time to become stronger and accommodate to the new workload soon to be imposed on them, so that the injuries that result from fatigue—patellofemoral compression, stress fractures, or plantar fasciitis—can be prevented.

In addition to lower-extremity strengthening, upper-body strengthening of both the trunk and the upper extremities is vital in runners, as has recently been stressed by Anderson [6].

Stretching

Stretching is vital to any training program, particularly in track. Just as it is necessary in the recovery phase from existing injury, it also is vital to prevent injury.

Improved muscle-tendon compliance is the goal in both the stretching and strengthening programs. The negative work theory of either isometric or eccentric contraction can be exploited to enhance the efficiency of functioning muscle-tendon units. Throwers, jumpers, and weight lifters can improve their performances by maximizing the characteristics of elastic recoil of their muscles and tendons. Training these components by appropriate stretching techniques allows for greater deformity of the muscle-tendon unit just before the abrupt shortening fundamental to throwing, jumping, or lifting. The result of stretched muscle suddenly shortened is superior force, power, and performance. In addition, enhanced flexibility from stretching will give greater muscle-tendon compliance. For any given load, greater compliance will allow greater muscle deformity and subsequent recoil.

Current concepts of stretching take into account newer neurophysiologic principles. The outmoded ballistic stretching technique—quick, jerky movement in an attempt to stretch the muscle or tendon—fails to accomplish its goal. The sudden stretch initiates a stretch reflex and subsequent muscle contraction. Shortening is the result. Even static stretching—gradual lengthening of the muscle group to its maximal length while carefully avoiding any muscle activity, thereby eliminating reflex stimulation of muscle—will fail if that stretch reflex is initiated.

Current neurophysiologic concepts suggest the use of central mechanisms to achieve maximal muscle-tendon length [7], the technique now preferred for stretching. Proprioceptive neuromuscular facilitation, originally devised by Kabat [8], employs reciprocal muscle innervation in addition to stretching the involved muscle-tendon unit. Specifically, the muscles are lengthened gradually with simultaneous isometric contraction of their agonist, to produce maximal relaxation of the muscles being stretched and prevent the initiation of the competing stretch reflex.

Holt has modified this technique in his 3S (Scientific Stretching for Sport) concept [9], citing improvements of increased joint motion, increased muscle-tendon flexibility, and increased muscle strength. In Holt's technique, the muscle is contracted isometrically to its lengthened position, followed by concentric contraction of the agonist muscle group.

Stretching is vital in the aging athlete, when the tendons are less resilient and the muscles less contractile, but it is equally important in the young athlete. Muscles and tendons are most effective not with bulk but with the greatest compliance possible. Finally, if we remember only one aspect of the conditioning program, it is to allow adequate time for stretching.

References

1. James, S.L., Bates, B.T., Ostering, L.R.   Injuries to runners. *Am. J. Sports Med.* 6:40–50, 1978.

2. Larson, R.L., Cabaud, H.E., Slocum, D.B., et al.   The patellar compression syndrome: surgical treatment by lateral retinacular release. *Clin. Orthop.* 134:158–167, 1978.

3. Noble, H.B., Hajek, M.R., Porter, M.   Diagnosis and treatment of iliotibial band tightness in runners. *Physician Sportsmed.* 10:67-74, 1982.

4. Puddu, G., Ippolito, E., Postacchini, F.   A classification of Achilles tendon disease. *Am. J. Sports Med.* 4:145–150, 1976.

5. Clancy, W.G., Jr.   Tendinitis and plantar fasciitis. In D'Ambrosia, R., Drez, D., Jr. (eds.), *Prevention and Treatment of Running Injuries.* Thorofare, N.J.: C.B. Slack, Inc., 1982, pp. 77–78.

6. Anderson, J.L.   Running for fitness is fine, but more must be done. *New York Times*, October 24, 1982, section 5, p. 2.

7. Stanish, W.D.   Neurophysiology of stretching. In D'Ambrosia, R., Drez, D., Jr. (cds.), *Prevention and Treatment of Running Injuries.* Thorofare, N.J.: C.B. Slack, Inc., 1982, pp. 135–146.

8. Kabat, H.   Studies of neuromuscular dysfunction—the role of central facilitation in resortation of motor function in paralysis. *Arch. Phys. Med.* 33:521–533, 1952.

9. Holt, L.E.   *Scientific Stretching for Sport.* Sport Research Ltd., 1973.

10. Clancy, W.G., Jr., Neidhart, D., Brand, R.L.   Achilles tendinitis in runners: a report of five cases. *Am. J. Sports Med.* 4:46–57, 1976.

11. Fulkerson, J.P., Gossling, H.R.   Anatomy of the knee joint lateral retinaculum. *Clin. Orthop.* 153:183–188, 1980.

12. Leach, R.E.   Running injuries of the knee. In D'Ambrosia, R., Drez, D., Jr. (eds.), *Prevention and Treatment of Running Injuries.* Thorofare, N.J.: C.B. Slack, Inc., 1982, pp. 57–76.

13. Mann, R.A.   Biomechanics of running. In D'Ambrosia, R., Drez, D., Jr. (eds)., *Prevention and Treatment of Running Injuries.* Thorofare, N.J.: C.B. Slack, Inc., 1982, pp. 1–14.

14. McMahon, T.A., Greene, P.R.   Fast running tracks. *Sci. Am.* December 1980, pp. 148–163.

17 Injuries in the Football Sports

Lyle J. Micheli, M.D.

There are three different versions of football presently being played in most parts of North America. Gridiron football, the most popular, is played in both the United States and Canada but by slightly different rules. Soccer football or, more properly, Association football is growing rapidly in popularity, particularly among children of both sexes, in part because of its presumed safety and simplicity of playing skills. Rugby football, introduced more than a century ago but then transformed into gridiron football, is undergoing a rebirth in both the United States and Canada, primarily at the university and adult city club level. Gaelic football and Australian rules football, the two additional versions of football, have only limited popularity in North America.

These football games frequently are compared and contrasted by their respective proponents as to the playing skills required, fitness levels needed for or improved by these sports, and the relative risk of injury associated with playing each of these games [1, 2]. It is the purpose of this chapter to assess the relative risk of injury reported for these sports, injury patterns or trends suggested by these reports, and finally, steps that might be taken to alter these patterns.

Gridiron Football

Gridiron football, the national sport of the United States, has remained a controversial sport because of its relatively high rate of overall injury and its potential for severe injury to the head, neck, and knees. To some extent, the overall risk of injury appears to be a function of the age and size of the individuals playing the game. Studies of children's organized football, usually done under the auspices of the Pop Warner Foundation, have been reassuring [3]. The reported injury rate has been low, with few serious injuries. Roser and Clawson [4], in a study of children's football in Seattle, found a rate of injury of 3.2 percent and deemed this quite acceptable when compared with other children's sports. Two more recent studies suggest a high rate of injury in children's football and may represent a warning with respect to the potential for an increased degree of injury when somewhat larger and more aggressive children are exposed to more systematic coaching and training [5, 6].

[1]Pop Warner Foundation, Philadelphia, Pennsylvania.

Although the information about youth football is, on the whole, reassuring, there remains real reason for concern at the high school level. In one of the first surveys of high school football injuries, published in 1967, Garrahan [7] found a 20 percent rate of injury. More recent studies by Blythe and Mueller [8], of North Carolina high school football, and Garrick and Requa [9], in Seattle, have found a significantly higher rate of overall injury, further suggesting that there is cause for concern.

Studies of injury rates at the college and professional football level have shown a relative consistency. Rates of injury at the college level range from 40 to 54 percent, and generally, it is accepted that professional football teams have a rate of 100 percent or more injured players per season [10, 11]. These statistics are becoming much more reproducible now that both the collegiate and professional football associations compile their injury records through the National Athletic Injury/Illness Reporting System (NAIRS) at Pennsylvania State University.[2]

Head and Neck Injuries

Somewhat more reassuring are recent reports regarding the occurrence of catastrophic head and neck injuries in football. Dr. Joseph Torg's initial report [12], published in 1979, found that 259 cervical spine fractures or dislocations occurred in organized football between 1971 and 1975. Similarly, in 1975, Albright et al. [13] reported a surprisingly high incidence of neck complaints and radiographic changes suggestive of preexistent injury in freshman football players at the University of Iowa. Both studies indicted techniques of butt blocking or spearing, in particular, as being associated with this unacceptable level of head and neck injury.

Another factor thought to be associated with head and neck injuries was the development of the hard-shell plastic football helmet and, more recently, the face mask. It has been suggested that the development of hard-shell helmets may well have decreased the incidence of cerebral injuries and concussions in football but, in so doing, may have increased the risk of neck injury by encouraging these better-protected players to strike opponents directly with the crown of the head while blocking or tackling [14]. That this piece of protective equipment for the head enhanced the risk of catastrophic neck injury is further suggested by Blythe's study [8], which found that the football helmet was the risk factor most frequently associated with all types of football injuries, including hip and thigh contusions and knee injuries.

The two approaches most frequently suggested to help resolve this serious problem were a change of helmet design (to a semirigid helmet, for

---

[2]NAIRS compiles intercollegiate and interscholastic injury or illness data reported by team trainers, physicians, and other health care personnel.

instance) and prohibition of the tactic of spearing and butt blocking. Albright et al. [13] even suggested barring the use of face masks, because they appear to be associated with an increased risk of neck injuries. To date, no serious changes in helmet design have evolved, but it appears that the tactic of spearing is being used less frequently in most parts of the country, particularly at the high school level, as a result of better coaching and officiating. More recent reports from Torg (personal communication) and the University of Iowa [15] are reassuring. Torg and Albright et al. have found a progressive decrease in the incidence of serious neck injury over the past 7 years. Whether this trend will continue and be further improved by changes in the helmet or face mask design remains to be seen.

Knee Injuries

Reports regarding knee injuries in gridiron football are not as reassuring. The *National Football Injury Report, 1970* [10] found an overall injury rate of 52 percent in college football, with the highest number of injuries occurring at the knee. Subsequent reports on football injuries from NAIRS have shown some fluctuations in the overall rate of injury from football, but the knee remains the leading site of injury.

Improvements in the overall conditioning of football players, including the widespread use of resistive weight training, has appeared to decrease this injury rate. Cahill [16] found a decreased incidence of knee injuries in high school players on weight training regimens and suggested that this was due to increased strength of the ligaments of the knee and increased strength of muscles and tendons, thus decreasing the chance of injury to these structures. It has been suggested that, though the bones and ligaments may indeed be stronger as a result of this weight training, the increased force of impact and intensity of play from these bigger, stronger players may more than compensate for the stronger tissues and explain the consistently high instance of serious knee injuries, particularly at the collegiate level.

A recent suggestion aimed at decreasing the incidence of knee injuries is the use of prophylactic knee bracing, particularly for high-risk positions such as interior lineman and running back. The apparatus that has been used most widely is the McDavid brace, which is attached to the lateral aspect of the knee. Anecdotal reports are encouraging, and the device is used routinely at such major universities as Notre Dame, but no published data are available yet to confirm the efficacy of this approach in decreasing injury.

Another suggested approach is attributable to Dr. T.R. Peterson [17], of Michigan, who has indicated the tactic of cross-body blocking as a source of a high proportion of serious knee injuries in football. A change of game rules at the high school and collegiate level has limited the use of this technique, and subsequent studies by Peterson suggest that there has been an associated decrease in ligamentous injuries to the knee. However, much more study of the relationship of football tactics to this continued source of serious injury is needed [18].

Soccer Football

Injuries in soccer football have proved to be very much a function of the age, skills, and even the sex of the participants. At the child and youth level, the reported incidence of injury has been low. A review of soccer injuries in Oklahoma found 7 injuries per 100 participants older than 12 years per season and 1 injury per 100 players younger than 12 per season, but girls were injured twice as frequently as boys [19]. Reports of soccer-related injuries in Europe at the schoolboy level now are available and suggest a very low rate of injury in well-coached and conditioned school-aged players [20].

The general pattern of injuries encountered in soccer football is primarily of the lower extremities, with knee injuries leading the list while ligamentous sprains about the foot and ankle run a close second [21]. Fortunately, these soccer knee injuries are less severe than those sustained in gridiron football; many of them are noncontact or cutting injuries. It has been suggested, however, that the relative occurrence of posterior cruciate ligament injuries is higher in soccer than in many other sports in the United States, due to hyperextension of the knee from blows to the front and inner aspect of the lower leg. The physician assessing a knee injury in a soccer player should be well aware of this.

Quadriceps contusions and muscle-tendon strains also are cited often in reviews of soccer injuries. Smodlaka's study [2] of adult and professional soccer players found a high incidence of musculotendinous injuries, particularly strains of the muscles spanning two joints, such as the hamstrings, quadriceps, and gastrocnemius, and suggested that systematic stretching programs might be valuable in decreasing the incidence of these injuries.

One of the frequently voiced concerns of observers of North American soccer programs is that inexperienced coaching and officiating persistently contributes not only to poor quality of play but also to increased risk of injury from a general low level of playing skills. Gross [22] found a widespread concern among American youth soccer coaches regarding their lack of coaching and training knowledge. Fortunately, the American Youth Soccer Foundation is well aware of this problem and is actively conducting workshops designed to improve coaching knowledge and skills. This would appear to be the single most effective step toward increasing the safety of North American soccer at this time.

Rugby Football

The game of rugby football, direct forerunner of gridiron football in the United States, is undergoing a widespread revival in North America. Rugby football and American football frequently are compared and contrasted by their respective proponents in terms of playing skills required and the relative danger involved in playing each sport. Unlike American gridiron football, which has evolved significantly, rugby football as presently played remains very similar to the early rugby style of play. In rugby football, there are 15 men per team and the game is divided into two 40-minute halves with no time-outs or substitutions allowed. Protective equipment, developed to a sophisticated and sometimes dangerous degree in American gridiron football, is specifically prohibited in rugby football.

The game begins with the kickoff. Play is continuous, except for stops for infractions of the rules, and running is the prime method of advancing the ball, although it can be kicked directly forward at any time by the ball carrier. An opponent carrying the ball may be tackled, but no blocking is allowed. The ball may be passed only laterally or backward. Any member of the team is eligible to receive a pass or field a kick. A team scores by running the ball across the goal line and touching it down, by kicking it through the uprights, or by a penalty kick.

Contributors to Injury Incidence

One of the less fortunate aspects of American rugby football is that many of its participants have previously been gridiron football players, and they often employ tactics that, although appropriate in gridiron football, are a potential source of injury in rugby. In particular, hitting with the head while attempting a tackle has been indicted in a number of serious rugby injuries.

Rugby football in this country is played primarily at the college or city club level. The fairly informal nature of the game in this country has tended to delay the development of systematic coaching and consistent refereeing. This lack of good coaching and officiating in games remains one of the major contributors to injury in rugby football in the United States. Ironically, even when played under the rather primitive conditions of unskilled players and sometimes dangerous tactics, rugby still is relatively safer than gridiron football.

A 1974 study showed an overall rate of injury of 9.8 percent in one season in the Boston area [1]. Other European investigators also have found a low rate of injury in this game, although it is characterized by many people as being more brutal than American gridiron football [23]. It is noteworthy that many of the injuries occurring in rugby football are of relatively minor severity, consisting of head and face lacerations and contusions, similar to hockey. The absence of body blocking, especially, appears to be one of the primary reasons for this lower rate of injury. In addition, when properly performed, the rugby tackle is very different from the American gridiron football tackle, insofar as the object is to capture the ball from the opponent rather than to knock the opponent down and prevent his or her linear progression on the field.

Head and Neck Injuries

One cause of serious concern in recent years is the apparent increased incidence of catastrophic head and neck injuries in rugby football. A study in Britain ascribed a significant number of these injuries to the collapsing of the scrummage, a play in which the forwards of each team meet head to head and the stronger team drives over the weaker team; in so doing, the front-row forwards sustain hyperflexion at the neck [24]. Steps to be taken to prevent this serious injury include systematic strengthening of the head, neck, and shoulder muscles of the front-row forwards, proper coaching in scrummage technique, and careful officiating with early detection of a tendency toward collapsing of the scrummage.

Knee and Shoulder Injuries

The two other major sites of injury in rugby are the knee and the shoulder. As with the other nonblocking football games, knee injuries can occur simply from cutting (i.e., changing directions quickly), with injuries to ligaments including the anterior cruciate ligament, and also as a result of direct blows in such loose action as the loose scrummage or maul. In American rugby, serious knee injuries often are the result of illegal or illogical tactics such as cross-body blocking or striking opponents low and hard when it would have been more logical to strike higher and attempt to obtain the ball. Once again, proper coaching can prevent this.

The high incidence of shoulder injuries, particularly acromioclavicular separations, is ascribed to a number of different mechanisms. Shoulder injuries can result from a tackle, a falling on the point of the shoulder, or falling on the outstretched arm in avoiding a tackle. An observer of the Irish rugby scene, Dr. T.J.C. O'Connell [25] at one point suggested a modified simple shoulder protector for the rugby shirt itself, but this would appear to be only a partial solution to the problem of shoulder injuries, especially those indirect injuries to the shoulder mechanism. Proper coaching can be useful in teaching tactics that avoid injury. The hardness of the playing surface is another very important factor in the incurrence of such injuries.

The Changing Face of Rugby

As noted previously, the greatest need in a relatively informal game such as rugby football is that of systematic coaching and officiating. This is rendered more difficult because of a lack of a school structure around which to organize coaching sessions or referee seminars.

The increased numbers of women's teams participating in rugby may ultimately be beneficial for the game. The women's style of playing, which is rapidly improving, does not emphasize high-impact hitting as does the men's game. Women have not had the disadvantage of previous exposure to gridiron football and, as a result, often play rugby football in a more logical fashion without unnecessary body contact or impact. In the early years of women's rugby in the Boston area, most injuries that we observed were of the overuse type, the result of lack of preparedness for running, twisting, or throwing. As this population of athletes has become progressively better conditioned to the demands of the game, the incidence of injuries has decreased significantly, and the incidence of high-impact traumatic injuries appears to remain much lower than in the men's game.

References

1. Micheli, L.J., Riseborough, E.J.   The incidence of injuries in rugby football. *Am. J. Sports Med.* 2:93–98, 1974.

2. Smodlaka, V.N.   Rehabilitation of injured soccer players. *Physician Sportsmed.* 7:59–67, 1979.

3. Godshall, R.W.   Junior league football: risks vs. benefits. *J. Sports Med. Phys. Fitness* 3:139–144, 1975.

4. Roser, L.A., Clawson, D.K.   Football injuries in the very young athlete. *Clin. Orthop.* 69:212–223, 1970.

5. Nettles, J.L.   Football related epiphyseal injuries. *Curr. Concepts Trauma Care,* 2:18–20, 1981.

6. Silverstein, B.M.   Injuries in youth league football. *Physician Sportsmed.* 9:105–113, 1979.

7. Garrahan, W.F.   Incidence of high school football injuries. *R.I. Med. J.* 50:833–835, 1967.

8. Blythe, C.S., Mueller, F.O.   Football injury survey: P + I. When and where players get hurt. *Physician Sportsmed.* 2:45–52, 1974.

9. Garrick, J.G., Requa, R.K.   Injuries in high school sports. *J. Pediatr.* 61:465–469, 1978.

10. Joint Commission on Competitive Safeguards and Medical Aspects of Sports.   *National Football Injury Report, 1970.* Lincoln: University of Nebraska, 1972.

11. Shields, C.L., Zomar, V.D.   Analysis of professional football injuries. *Contemp. Orthop.* 4:90–95, 1982.

12. Torg, J.S., Quedenfeld, T.C., Burstein, A., et al.   National football head and neck injury registry: report on cervical quadriplegia, 1971–1975. *Am. J. Sports Med.* 7:127–132, 1979.

13. Albright, J.P., Moses, J.M., Feldrick, H.G., et al.   Non-fatal cervical spine injuries in interscholastic football. *J.A.M.A.* 236:1243–1245, 1976.

14. Schneider, R.C.   Serious and fatal neurosurgical football injuries. *Clin. Neurosurg.* 12:226–236, 1966.

15. Albright, J.P., Crowley, E., Foster, D., et al.   Patterns of Nonfatal Neck Injuries in Iowa Football: A Nine Year Experience. Paper presented at the Interim Meeting of the American Orthopedics Society for Sports Medicine, Anaheim, Calif., 1983.

16. Cahill, B.R.   Pre-season Conditioning in Football. Paper presented to the American Orthopedics Society for Sports Medicine, San Diego, 1977.

17. Peterson, T.R.   The cross body block, the major cause of knee injuries. *J.A.M.A.* 211:449–452, 1970.

18. Peterson, T.R. Rule changes at the high school and collegiate level. Paper presented at the Meeting of the American Orthopedics Society for Sports Medicine, Lake Tahoe, Nevada, 1981.

19. Sullivan, J.A., Gross, R.H., Grana, W.A., et al.   Evaluation of injuries in youth soccer. *Am. J. Sports Med.* 8:325–327, 1980.

20. Nilsson, S., Roaas, A.   Soccer injuries in adolescents. *Am. J. Sports Med.* 6:358–361, 1978.

21. Ekstrand, J., Gillquist, J., Moller, M., et al.   Incidence of soccer injuries and their relations to training and team success. *Am. J. Sports Med.* 11:63–67, 1983.

22. Gross, R.H.   Training programs for volunteer coaches: more time, more money. *Physician Sportsmed.* 10:183–185, 1982.

23. Archibald, R.M.   An analysis of rugby football injuries in the 1961–62 season. *Practitioner* 189:333–334, 1962.

24. Scher, A.T.   Rugby injuries to the cervical spinal cord. *S. Afr. Med. J.* 51(14):473–475, 1977.

25. O'Connell, T.C.J.   Rugby football injuries and their prevention. *J. Irish Med. Assoc.* 34:20–26, 1954.

Index

Abdominal paradox, 143
Achilles tendinitis, 195–196
  causes of, 195
  treatment of, 195–196
Acromioclavicular joint, 180, 184
Adductor magnus muscle, in sculling,
  174–175
Age
  cross-country skiing performance
    study of, 17, 18–19
  developmental, determination of, 3–4
  performance, determination of, 4
American Athletic Association for the
  Deaf (AAAD), 36
American Blind Bowling Association,
  34–35
American Coalition of Citizens with
  Disabilities, 40
American College of Sports Medicine
  (ACSM), 94
American Thoracic Society (ATS), 139,
  144, 149
American Youth Soccer Foundation, 206
Amputees. See also Handicapped sports
  sports available to, 29, 30, 31–32
  sports organizations for, 37–40
Anaerobic threshold
  cardiopulmonary exercise testing
    with, 112
  exercise prescription and, 94
  rating of perceived exertion (RPE)
    and, 101
  ventilatory responses in exercise
    testing with, 116, 118, 120–121
Ankle injuries, in baseball, 179
Antiinflammatory agents, 185, 186, 194
Anxiety, and hypotension after exer-
  cise, 130–132
Archer, Ken, 33
Archery, 40
Arm ergometry (A), ventilatory respon-
  ses to, 115–125
Arthrography, in shoulder injury, 184
Aspirin, 185, 186

Baseball
  body structures injured most often
    in, 179, 181

Children's Hospital Medical Center
  (Boston) experience with injuries
  in, 179, 180
Dizzy Dean syndrome in, 179–180
injury prevention and rehabilitation
  in, 179–190
Little League elbow in, 188–189
pitcher's shoulder in, 181
players most vulnerable to injury in,
  179
playing with injuries in, 179–180
shoulder injury in, 180–186
sports talent in children for, 10
Basketball, wheelchair. See Wheelchair
  basketball
Behavior coaching, 73–91
  behavior analysis in, 83
  behavior prescription in, 87, 88
  client's style of relating to coach in,
    82
  coach as role model in, 85
  data gathering in, 81–84
  description of, 77–78
  follow-up visits in, 86
  general principles of, 79–81
  health psychology in, 76–79
  history taking in, 82–83
  impact of change on other people
    of, 88–89
  as intervention, 79
  life-style/health relationships in, 73–76
  macrosocial contexts of, 89–90
  microsocial contexts of, 87–89
  psychosocial history in, 83
  punishment in, 86
  reinforcement and feedback in, 81,
    85–86
  social system and support network
    in, 78–79, 87–88
  strategic intervention in, 84–87
Behavior modification, 77
Bench press power output study. See
  Power output study
Beta-blocker medication, and hypotension after exercise, 129, 130, 133,
  134, 136
Bicycle ergometry (B), and ventilatory
  responses to, 115–125

211

Biomechanical considerations, 161–175
  electromyographic analysis of scull-
    ing, 169–175
  power outputs at areas of range of
    motion, 163–167
Blind. *See also* Handicapped sports
  skiing by, 63, 65–66
  sports organizations for, 34–35
Blind Outdoors Leisure Development,
  35
Blood pressure, and exercise, 109, 129
Body composition
  choice of sport in children and,
    7–9
  in cross-country skiing performance
    study, 16, 17, 18–19, 20–21
  mask-flippers-snorkel (MFS) exer-
    cise program and, 55, 57
  in wheelchair basketball study,
    46–47, 48, 50
Boston Marathon, 32–33
Bowling, handicapped, 34–35
Bracing, knee, 206
Breathing exercises
  inspiratory muscle training (IMT),
    147–149
  intermittent positive pressure breath-
    ing (IPPB), 144–145
  in pulmonary rehabilitation, 146–
    149
Breathing patterns, in chronic obstruc-
    tive pulmonary disease (COPD),
    142–143
Bronchodilators, 144–145

Camping, for handicapped, 40–41
Cardiac disorders, and mask-flippers-
    snorkel (MFS) exercise program,
    55–60
Cardiac function tests, in mask-flippers-
    snorkel (MFS) exercise program,
    55, 59, 60. *See also* Cardiopul-
    monary exercise testing
Cardiopulmonary considerations, 107–
    160
  exercise testing and, 109–114
  and hypotension after exercise
    study, 129–137
  and rehabilitation of pulmonary
    patient, 139–156
  ventilatory responses to exercise
    modalities, 115–125

Cardiopulmonary exercise testing, 109–
    114
  clinical applicability of data from,
    125
  clinical reasons for, 109
  diagnostic uses of, 113–114
  differences between men and
    women in, 124–125
  disability evaluation with, 113
  measurements included in, 109–113
  methods in study of, 115–116
  normal values in, 113
  results in study of, 116–118
  types of exercises used in, 115
  ventilatory responses to, 115–125
Carter, Jimmy, 89
Cheff Center for the Handicapped, 31
Chest physical therapy techniques,
    145–146
Children
  body composition profile in, 7–9
  chin-up tests in, 5–6
  choice of sport by, 3–13
  developmental age determination in,
    3–4
  endurance tests in, 7
  fifty-yard sprint in, 5
  flexibility performance tests in,
    8, 9, 10
  football injuries in, 203
  height in, 8
  hopscotch performance test in, 6, 7
  leg and trunk length in, 8, 9
  Little League elbow in, 188–189
  muscle profile tests in, 4–6
  neurologic profile in, 6–7
  performance age determination in, 4
  ruler drop performance test in, 6–7
  vertical jump tests in, 4–5
Chin-up tests, in children's choice of
    sport, 5–6, 12
Chondromalacia, 68, 179
Chronic obstructive pulmonary disease.
    See Pulmonary disease, chronic
    obstructive (COPD)
Cold injury, in handicapped skiing,
    69–70
Competition, in handicapped sports,
    31, 32–33, 68
Cornell Adult Fitness Program, 101
Coronary artery disease, 75
Cough, in pulmonary rehabilitation, 146

Cross-country skiing
  data collection in study of, 16–17
  lean body weight (LBW) in, 16,
    20–21
  performance prediction study in,
    15–22
  physical work capacity (PWC) in,
    16–17, 20–21, 22
  results of performance study in,
    17–21
  sports talent in children for, 10
  variables in, 16
Cruciate ligament injuries, 206, 208

Dance sports, and ability in children, 12
Deaf, sports organizations for, 36–37.
    See also Handicapped; Han-
    dicapped skiing; Handicapped
    sports
Decathlon, 13
Depression, 156
Diaphragm, in pulmonary rehabilita-
    tion, 140–141
Disabled. See Handicapped sports
Diuretic medication, and hypotension
    after exercise, 129, 130, 133,
    135–136
Dizzy Dean syndrome, 179–180
Downhill skiing, 10
Drug therapy
  elbow injuries in baseball with, 185,
    186
  running injuries and, 194

Eating patterns, and health, 75
Education
  health and, 76
  in pulmonary rehabilitation pa-
    tients, 156
Elbow injuries, in baseball, 179, 186–
    190
  anatomy of elbow in, 186, 187
  Little League elbow in, 188–189
  overuse syndromes in, 186–189
  sprain in, 186
  throwing mechanisms and, 187
  treatment of, 189
Electrocardiography (ECG), in cardio-
    pulmonary exercise testing, 110
Electromyography analysis in sculling.
    See Sculling electromyography
    (EMG) study

Endurance tests, and sports ability in
    children, 7
Exercise prescription, 93–103
  guidelines for, 102
  heart rate as predictor of oxygen
    consumption in, 94–95
  oxygen consumption in, 93–94
  rating of perceived exertion (RPE)
    in, 95–103
Exercise programs. See also Cardio-
    pulmonary exercise testing
  changes expected with, 155
  evaluation scales in, 151
  for handicapped, 33–34, 67
  intensity, frequency, and duration
    of, 151–155
  lateral patellar compression syn-
    drome with, 194
  mask-flippers-snorkel (MSF) aquatic
    therapeutic, 53–60
  oxygen use in, 155
  power output studies and, 166–167
  pulmonary rehabilitation with, 149–
    155
  running injury prevention with,
    199–200
Exercise testing, wheelchair basketball
    study with, 47–51. See also Car-
    diopulmonary exercise testing
Exertion. See Rating of perceived exer-
    tion (RPE)

Feedback, in behavior coaching, 81,
    85–86
Fifty-yard sprint, and athletic ability in
    children, 5
Figure skating, 12
Fishing, handicapped, 31, 32
Flexibility performance tests, and athletic
    ability in children, 8, 9, 10, 12, 13
Football, 203–209
  athletic ability in children and, 11,
    12
  contributors to injury incidence in,
    207–209
  gridiron, 203–206
  head and neck injuries in, 204–205,
    208
  helmet design in, 204–205
  knee injuries in, 205–206, 208
  risk of injuries in, 203
  women's teams in, 209

Foot injuries, in baseball, 179
Forced expiratory volume in one second (FEV₁), 110
Four-track skiing, 64
Fractures. *See* Stress fractures

Gardening, for handicapped, 41
Gastrocnemius muscle, in sculling, 172–173
Glenohumeral joint, 180
Gluteus maximus muscle, in sculling, 175
Gridiron football injuries, 203–206
Gymnastics, 10

Hall, Bob, 32–33
Handicapped
    conditions included in, 27
    fitness for, 27–43
    need for recreational activity by, 27
    physiology of exercise for, 28
    public attitudes toward, 28
Handicapped skiing, 29, 63–70
    cold injury in, 69–70
    competition and racing in, 68, 69
    equipment used in, 64–65
    fatigue and thigh burn in, 70
    four-track skiing in, 64
    instructional methods and sequence in, 65–66, 66–67, 68
    knee problems and, 68–69
    lower-extremity amputation or weakness and, 63–65
    organizations for, 35, 37, 38, 66
    outriggers in, 29, 64, 70
    physical assessment in, 63–66
    program sites in, 63, 67
    sit-skiing in, 65
    special risks for, 68–70
    tri-track skiing in, 64, 67
    visual impairment in, 65–66
    warm-up before, 69
Handicapped sports, 25–70
    availability of, 29–32
    benefits of, 27, 28
    bibliography of, 40–43
    competition opportunities in, 32–33
    exercise programs in, 33–34
    historical perspectives on, 27–28

lower-limb-disabled recreational pursuits in, 33, 35
mask-flippers-snorkel (MFS) exercise program in, 53–60
organizations for, 34–40
selection of, 28–33
skiing in, 63–70
special considerations in, 28–29
upper- and lower-limb-disabled pursuits in, 33, 36
upper-limb-disabled pursuits in, 33, 34
Head injuries, in football, 204–205, 208
Health
    health psychology applied to, 76
    life-style and, 73–76
Health care system, 89–90, 91
Health psychology, 76–79
    behavior coaching and, 77–79
    definition of, 76–77
Heart rate, and oxygen consumption, 94–95
Heart tests. *See* Cardiopulmonary exertion tests
Height
    choice of sport in children and, 8, 13
    cross-country skiing performance study and, 17, 18–19
Helmets, football, 204–205
Hoover's sign, 143
Hopscotch performance test, 6, 7, 12
Horseback riding, and handicapped, 30–31, 37–38, 39
Hypotension after exercise (study), 129–137
    beta-blocker medication in, 129, 130, 133, 134, 146
    diuretic medication in, 129, 130, 133, 135–136
    intervention protocols in, 132–133
    methods used in, 129–132
    results of, 133–136
    self-reported anxiety levels in, 130–132
    subjects in, 129

Ice hockey, 11, 12
Iliotibial band friction syndrome, 194, 199
Illinois Sport Competition Anxiety Test (SCAT), 15, 16, 17, 20–21

Illness
  health psychology applied to, 76
  life-style and, 74–76
Injury prevention, 177–210
  baseball, 179–190
  football, 203–209
  track, 193–200
Inspiratory muscle training (IMT),
  147–149
Intermittent positive pressure breathing
  (IPPB), 144–145
International Committee of the Silent
  Sports, 36–37
International Organization for the
  Disabled, 32

Joint problems, handicapped skiing
  and, 68–69. See also Elbow injuries; Knee injuries; Shoulder
  injuries

Knee injuries
  in baseball, 179
  conditioning and bracing for, 205
  football and, 205–206, 208
  handicapped skiing and, 68–69
  iliotibial band friction syndrome in,
    194
  lateral patellar compression syn-
    drome in, 193–194
  strengthening exercises in running
    and, 194, 199

Lateral patellar compression syndrome,
  193–194, 198
Lean body weight (LBW), in cross-
  country skiing performance
  study, 16, 17, 18–19, 20–21
Leg length, and athletic ability in children, 8, 9
Life-style, and health, 73–76
Ligament injuries, in baseball, 179,
  181
Little League elbow, 188–189
Lung capacity, athletic ability in children and, 9, 11, 13. See also
  Cardiopulmonary considerations;
  Cardiopulmonary exercise
  testing; Pulmonary disease,
  chronic obstructive; Pulmonary
  function tests; Pulmonary
  rehabilitation

Marathons, 32–33
Mask-flippers-snorkel (MFS) aquatic
  therapeutic exercise program,
  53–60
  and cardiac and orthopedic dis-
    orders, 55–60
  cardiac tests in, 55, 59, 60
  instruction in, 54
  methods of study of, 54
  origination of, 53–54
  pulmonary function tests and, 55,
    58, 60
  results of study of, 55
  subjects in study of, 55, 56
Maximal voluntary ventilation (MVV),
  110
Monollel skiing, 67
Muscles. See also Power output
    study
  baseball injuries and, 179, 191
  chronic obstructive pulmonary dis-
    ease (COPD) and, 142–143
  elbow injuries in baseball and, 186
  mechanism of throwing and, 183
  profiles of, in children's choice of
    sport, 4–6
  sculling electromyography (EMG)
    of, 169–175
  shoulder injury in baseball and,
    180, 182
  stretching exercises in running and,
    199–200

National Athletic Injury/Illness Reporting Service (NAIRS), 204,
  205
National Foundation for Happy Horsemanship for the Handicapped,
  37–38
National Handicapped Sports and Recreational Association, 38
National Wheelchair Athletic Association (Handicapped) (NWAA), 38
National Wheelchair Basketball Association, 38–39
National Wheelchair Games and International Paralympics, 32
Neck injuries, in football, 204–205,
  208
Neuritis, ulnar, 189
Neurologic profile, and athletic ability
  in children, 6–7

New England Handicapped Sportsman's Association, 63, 66
Nordic skiing. *See* Cross-country skiing
North American Riding for the Handicapped Association, 39
Nutrition, in pulmonary rehabilitation, 156

Obesity, 75, 113, 156
Organizations, for handicapped sports, 34–40, 66
Orthopedic disorders, and mask-flippers-snorkel (MFS) exercise program, 53, 55–60
Outriggers, in handicapped sports, 29, 64, 70
Overuse syndrome
    definition of, 182
    diagnosis of, 184–185
    elbow injuries in, 186–189
    football injuries in, 209
    running injuries in, 193–197
    shoulder injury in baseball in, 181–186
    treatment of, 185–186
Oxygen consumption
    anaerobic threshold in, 94
    assay methods in, 111
    cardiopulmonary exercise testing and, 111, 112
    cross-country skiing performance study of, 17, 18–19, 20, 21
    diagnostic uses of, 113–114
    exercise programs and, 93–94, 155
    heart rate as predictor of, 94–95
    rating of perceived exertion (RPE) with, 96–97, 98–100, 101
    wheelchair basketball study of, 50
Oxygen pulse, in cardiopulmonary exercise testing, 112–113

Pain, in running injuries, 198
Panner's disease, 188
Paraplegics, and sports choice, 29, 30
Patellar compression syndrome, 193–194
Patient education, in pulmonary rehabilitation, 156
Perceived exertion. *See* Rating of perceived exertion (RPE)
Peformance age, determination of, 4

Performance prediction, 1–22
    children's choice of sport with, 3–13
    cross-country skiing and, 15–22
Physical work capacity (PWC), in cross-country skiing performance study, 16–17, 20–21, 22
Pitcher's shoulder, 181
Plantar fasciitis, 196–197
Power output study, 163–167
    conditions for, 164
    custom training programs and, 166–167
    methods in, 163–164
    results of, 164–167
Psychological considerations, 71–105
    in behavior coaching, 73–91
    prescription of exercise and, 93–103
Psychosocial evaluation scales, in pulmonary rehabilitation, 144
Psychosocial support, in pulmonary rehabilitation, 155–156
Puberty, in developmental age determination, 3–4
Public attitudes, toward handicapped, 28
Public education, and health, 76
Pulmonary disease, chronic obstructive (COPD), 141
    breathing exercises in, 146–149
    bronchodilators in, 145
    chest physical therapy techniques in, 145–146
    evaluation tools in, 143–144
    exercise training in, 149–155
    Hoover's sign in, 143
    intermittent positive pressure breathing (IPPB) in, 145
    muscle fatigue and respiratory failure in, 142–143
    patient education on, 156
    physical examination in, 142
    physiologic alterations in, 141–142
Pulmonary function tests. *See also* Cardiopulmonary exercise testing
    mask-flippers-snorkel (MFS) exercise programs with, 55, 58, 60
    and wheelchair basketball study, 47, 48, 50
Pulmonary rehabilitation, 139–156
    breathing exercises in, 146–149
    bronchodilators in, 144–145

bronchopulmonary hygiene in, 144–146

chest physical therapy techniques in, 145–146

components of, 139

cough in, 146

definition of, 139

diaphragm in, 140–141

evaluation tools in, 143–144

exercise training in, 149–155

Hoover's sign in, 143

intermittent positive pressure breathing (IPPB) in, 144–145

muscle fatigue and respiratory failure in, 142–143

nutrition in, 156

patient education in, 156

patient selection in, 140

physiologic alterations in COPD and, 141–142

psychosocial support in, 155–156

pulmonary, physical, and psychosocial examination in, 140–144

therapy program formulation in, 144–145

Quadriceps muscles
lateral patellar compression syndrome and, 194
sculling and, 170–171, 175
soccer football injuries to, 206

Quadriplegics, and breathing patterns, 143

Racing
cross-country skiing performance in, 15–22
handicapped skiing and, 68, 69

Rating of perceived exertion (RPE), in exercise prescription, 95–103
criticism of, 101
oxygen consumption in, 96–97, 98–100, 101
physiologic basis of, 97
ratings scale used in, 95–96

Rectus abdominis muscle, in sculling, 174

Rehabilitation, definition of, 139. See also Pulmonary rehabilitation

Reinforcement, in behavior coaching, 81, 85–86

Respiratory alternans, 143

Riding, and handicapped, 30–31, 37–38, 39

Roentgenograms, in shoulder overuse syndrome, 184–185

Rugby football injuries, 203, 207–209

Ruler drop performance tests, 6–7, 12

Running
Achilles tendinitis in, 195–196
children's athletic talent for, 13
common injuries in, 193–197
handicapped and, 32–33
iliotibial band friction syndrome in, 194
injury analysis in, 197–198
injury prevention and rehabilitation in, 193–200
lateral patellar compression syndrome in, 193–194
pain and, 198
plantar fasciitis in, 196–197
posterior tibial tendinitis in, 196
rest or modification of routine in, 198–199
running conditions and injury in, 198
strengthening in, 199
stress fractures in, 197
stretching in, 199–200
training programs and injury in, 198

Sculling electromyography (EMG) study, 169–175
materials in, 169
protocol in, 169–170
results of, 170
stair climbing and descending study compared with, 172, 175
walking study compared with, 170–171, 175

Severely disabled. See Handicapped; Handicapped skiing; Handicapped sports

Sex differences in exercise testing, 124–125

Shoulder injuries, in baseball, 179, 180–186
anatomy of shoulder and, 180–181
diagnosis of, 184–185
mechanism of throwing and, 183–184
roentgenograms in, 184–185
shoulder overuse syndromes and, 181–186
treatment of, 185–186

Shoulder injuries, in football, 208
Sit-skiing, 65
Skiing. *See* Cross-country skiing; Handicapped skiing
Sky diving, 30
Soccer
   athletic ability in children for, 11, 12
   injuries in, 203, 206
Social system, and behavior coaching, 78–79, 88–89
Special Olympics, 39–40
Sport, children's choice of, 3–13
   bat and racquet sports in, 12
   body composition profile in, 7–9
   chin-up tests in, 5–6
   dance sports in, 12
   developmental age determination and, 3–4
   endurance tests in, 7
   fifty-yard sprint in, 5
   flexibility performance tests in, 8, 9, 10
   height in, 8
   hopscotch performance test in, 6, 7
   leg and trunk length in, 8, 9
   lung capacity in, 9, 11
   meaning and use of tests in, 9–10
   muscle profile in, 4–6
   neurologic profile in, 6–7
   performance age determination in, 4
   ruler drop performance test in, 6–7
   scoring tests in, 11
   swimming in, 12–13
   team field sports in, 11–12
   track and field sports in, 13
   types of tests for athletic talent in, 4–10
   vertical jump tests in, 4–5
Sport Competition Anxiety Test (SCAT), 15, 16, 17, 20–21
Sports activity, need for by handicapped, 27
Sprain, elbow, 186
Sprint swimming, 13
Steroids
   running injuries and, 195–196
   shoulder injury and, 186
Sternoclavicular joint, 180
Strengthening exercises, in running, 199
Stress fractures
   Little League elbow with, 188–189
   running and, 197

Stretching exercises, in running, 199–200
Support systems
   behavior coaching and, 78–79, 87–88
   in pulmonary rehabilitation, 155–156
Swimming
   children's athletic activity for, 10, 12–13
   handicapped and, 32, 42–43
   mask-flippers-snorkel (MFS) exercise program and, 53–60
   shoulder overuse syndrome in, 181

Target shooting, 31
Team field sports, and athletic talent in children, 11–12
Tendon injuries, in baseball, 179, 181
Tendinitis
   Achilles, 195–196
   posterior tibial, 196
Tendinosis, 195
Tennis, 12
   injuries in, 181, 186–187
Tenosynovitis, 195
Tenovaginitis, 195
Tests, for athletic talent in children, 4–11. *See also* Cardiopulmonary exercise testing; Exercise testing
Throwing mechanisms
   elbow injuries and, 187
   shoulder injury and, 183–184
Track. *See* Running
Track and field sports, and children's athletic ability, 13
Training programs. *See also* Exercise programs
   power output studies and, 166–167
   running injuries and, 198
   wheelchair basketball and, 45
Treadmill (T) exercise testing, ventilatory responses to, 115–125
Tri-track skiing, 64, 67
Trunk length, and athletic ability in children, 8, 9, 12, 13

United States Deaf Skiers Association, 37
U.S. National Wheelchair Games and International Paralympics, 32
United States Ski Association (USSA), 15

Vertical jump test, and athletic ability in children, 4–5, 12, 13
Visual impairment, skiing and, 64, 65–66. *See also* Blind; Handicapped sports

Walking
    handicapped and, 32
    sculling study compared with, 170–171, 175
Waterskiing, 29–30, 31
Water sports, and handicapped, 31, 43
Weight
    choice of sport by children and, 8
    lean body (LBW), in cross-country skiing performance study, 16, 17, 18–19, 20–21
    mask-flippers-snorkel (MFS) exercise program and, 55, 57

Weight training, and football injuries, 205
Wheelchair basketball, 45–51
    anthropometric changes in, 48, 50
    maximal oxygen uptake in, 50
    metabolic function changes in, 49, 51
    methods in study of, 46
    organization for, 38–39
    physiologic function changes in, 48–49, 50–51
    pulmonary function changes in, 48, 50
    results of study of, 48–49
    subjects in study of, 45–46
    test protocol in study of, 46-47
    training programs in, 45
Work load estimation, in cardiopulmonary exercise testing, 110